THE HAPPY BOWEL

First published 2018 by
FREMANTLE PRESS
25 Quarry Street, Fremantle WA 6160
(PO Box 158, North Fremantle WA 6159)
www.fremantlepress.com.au

Printed by McPherson's, Australia

 A catalogue record for this
book is available from the
National Library of Australia

The Happy Bowel. A user-friendly guide to bowel health for the whole family.
ISBN: 9781925591231 (paperback)

 Department of
**Local Government, Sport
and Cultural Industries**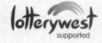
                              supported

Fremantle Press is supported by the State Government through the
Department of Local Government, Sport and Cultural Industries.

 **Australia
Council
for the Arts**

Publication of this title was assisted by the Commonwealth Government
through the Australia Council, its arts funding and advisory body.

THE HAPPY BOWEL

A user-friendly guide to bowel health for the whole family

Dr Michael Levitt MBBS, FRACS

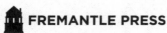 FREMANTLE PRESS

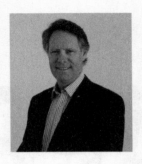

Dr Michael Levitt MBBS (UWA), FRACS trained as a surgeon in Western Australia before pursuing subspecialty training in colorectal surgery at London's St Mark's and Royal Free hospitals. Since 1990 he has worked in WA as a specialist colorectal surgeon. Michael has a particular interest in the management of 'functional' bowel disorders – constipation, incontinence and irritable bowel syndrome – and is well known for his approach to treating these conditions. Michael is a member of the Colorectal Surgical Society of Australia and New Zealand. He is the Chairman of the Tonkinson Colorectal Cancer Research Fund Advisory Committee, a Director of St John of God Health Care, a member of the Medical Board of WA and Medical Director at Osborne Park Hospital, WA. In 2003 Michael received a Centenary Medal in recognition of his work in raising public awareness and understanding about colorectal cancer. He has published several chapters in surgical textbooks and over 30 articles in peer-reviewed medical journals, and is the author of *The Bowel Book* (2002) and *The (Other) Women's Movement* (2008).

Contents

Introduction

On most days of their lives, a sizeable percentage of the human population of this planet opens their bowels. True, some do so with relatively less frequency or greater difficulty, while others do so more than once a day or with unseemly urgency. All in all, however, on every single day, throughout every corner of our planet, an innumerable number of human bowel actions takes place.

In the process of all this bowel opening, we humans can and do experience substantial stress and distress; failure and success; pleasure, agony and despair; anxiety, self-recrimination, frustration and exhaustion; satisfaction, pride, jubilation and even, occasionally, true wonder. The full gamut of these emotions will arise virtually every day for literally billions of people in the course of carrying out – or even just thinking about carrying out – an exercise that can take anything from a few desperate seconds to any number of interminable, lonely minutes.

Given the undeniably important role that opening our bowels plays in the broad sweep of human existence, it is truly mystifying that this pivotal bodily function enjoys such a diminutive place in our society. Rather than forming the basis of informed discussion, it is generally relegated to the dismal ranks of what is disparagingly referred to as 'toilet humour'. Even in the world of science, virtually all considered research is directed elsewhere.

It's true that there is inherent sensory offence associated with even the most ordinary of bowel actions. It's also true that other, more extraordinary bowel actions – often produced by otherwise unremarkable individuals – can result in memorably nauseating or unequivocally toxic emissions that inhibit clear thought, let alone dispassionate scientific discourse. Yet we are rarely offended by our own issue, however voluminous or malodorous it might be. Indeed, it is truly ironic that we can be physically repulsed by a fellow human being's defecatory efforts while remaining unmoved or even frankly impressed by our own entirely similar output.

There is, in fact, much about the use of our bowels and the impact this routine function has on our lives that is difficult to explain. But in the course of a career devoted to analysing and trying to improve the bowel habits of individuals puzzled and bedevilled by the malfunction and outright failure of their bowels, I have been able to identify many of the factors that can contribute to such failure and, likewise, to isolate the critical elements of a successful, satisfying bowel habit. There are indeed a few all-important Golden Rules for success, and associated clear guidelines for satisfaction, and together these can help us to achieve a happy bowel.

The purpose of this book is to introduce and explain these rules and guidelines, and to assist you in achieving happiness and relief in the course of using your bowel.

Michael Levitt
MBBS (UWA), FRACS

1

What's normal?

It's remarkable how often patients will describe their bowel habits to me as being 'normal' – as if they've conducted a thorough investigation into the bowel habits of a large and random sample of people of both sexes and all ages and found themselves to be situated comfortably within the mid-range. In truth, there is a very wide range of bowel habits among the general population, which means that at least some aspects of almost anyone's bowel habit could be described as normal.

In fact, what most people mean by describing their bowel habits as normal is generally quite straight-forward: as far as the average person is concerned, normal means having one bowel action every day.

There are people who believe that going more than once a day is a sign of exceptional normality, and regard such frequency as a desirable, even noble goal. There are others who think that regularity – having that all-important daily bowel action at the same time every day – is also normal, proudly announcing that they could 'set their clock' by the workings of their bowel, and feeling pleased and even righteous as a result. Others, still, attribute normality to bowel actions that float rather than sink; for these individuals, the relative buoyancy of their output appears to hold particular significance.

But by and large, most people are more or less of the opinion that 'normal' means 'daily'. However, while I can confirm that a daily bowel action is indeed approximately average for the human population as a whole (and I personally *have* conducted an investigation into the bowel functions of a large and random sample of people of both genders and all ages), this view of normality fails to acknowledge the wide range of variations that exist among us and – even worse – fails to recognise that a daily bowel action does not necessarily equate to a satisfactory bowel habit.

'Normal' versus satisfactory

Assessing the adequacy of a bowel habit on the basis of stool frequency alone completely ignores a whole range of factors that turn out to be vastly more important in determining whether we experience a truly satisfying bowel action or have a genuinely satisfactory bowel habit. And, as for regularity and buoyancy, these are of even less significance.

So what makes a bowel action 'satisfactory'? As it turns out, there are four key characteristics, which we'll take a look at now.

The four key characteristics of a satisfactory bowel action

In all of recorded human history, every truly satisfactory bowel action has had four things in common: it has been *prompt*, *effortless*, *brief* and *complete*. Wherever and by whomever it might have been produced, any human bowel action that has possessed all four of these characteristics will have represented a genuinely positive life experience for that person. And any individual who can say that they achieve such agreeable bowel actions on a majority of their visits to the bathroom can rightly claim to have a good bowel habit.

You need only ask yourself: 'Do I regularly commence rectal evacuation with a minimum of delay? Does it involve a minimum of effort? Am I regularly able to leave the bathroom after just a short period of time? And do I leave feeling satisfyingly empty?' If the answer to all of these questions is 'Yes', then you have an excellent bowel habit. If it's not, then you are likely to be struggling.

Notice that what does not count here – or, at least, not to anywhere near the same extent – is stool frequency, or how many times a day or a week you empty your bowel. This is an extremely important point: *How often you go is simply not as important as how easily and how completely you empty your bowel.*

People who are having difficulty with their bowels – those who are not able to experience the simple but significant pleasure of having regularly satisfactory bowel actions – can almost always describe their difficulty with reference to one or more of these four characteristics. They might experience delay with the initiation of bowel actions, difficulty getting bowel actions to pass, lengthy periods of time in the bathroom or an inability to completely empty their bowel. While many different factors and conditions can cause trouble with our bowels, they virtually all manifest as problems in one or more of these four key areas.

Throughout the course of this book you will see how these four potential sources of bowel trouble – initiation, effort, duration and completion – are all interrelated, and how difficulties in one area can often result in difficulties in the others. Before we move on, however, let's get out of the way two far less important characteristics that people are often (needlessly) concerned about.

What about odour and buoyancy?

Odour and buoyancy are two qualities of the output of our bowels that we all notice and perhaps sometimes wonder about but rarely discuss, so they are each worthy of brief discussion here.

Is it supposed to smell bad?

Odour is part and parcel of bowel function. Both the solid and the gaseous outputs of our bowels smell and, by common consensus, both of these smells are offensive – all the more so when they have been produced by someone else.

Given that we all eat food, and that most foods when left outside to rot will acquire an offensive odour, it shouldn't be too surprising that exactly those same sorts of foods, when mixed together and kept inside us at body temperature for 24 hours or more, will end up smelling bad. Add to this the smells associated with the gases produced by the action of the bacteria living in our bowels (more on this later), and there are good grounds for the output of our bowels to have an offensive odour.

Interestingly, the gases we produce in the largest quantities – hydrogen, carbon dioxide, methane, oxygen and nitrogen – are odourless. Much of this gas is derived from swallowed air and not necessarily from bacterial action in the bowel. This explains why the gas we produce is not always offensive and is, occasionally, entirely odourless. It is the sulphur-containing gases that primarily account for the offensive odour. The main gas in this group is hydrogen sulphide; others include methanethiol and dimethyl sulphide. Which particular foods contribute to the production of each specific gas is not, however, quite so clearly understood.

In fact, there is much that we do not yet know about the precise composition of the gases that emanate from our bowels. Recently there has been increased interest in the significance of the bacterial population of the human bowel, and how variations in this balance can affect our health. Even the fantastic notion of 'transplanting' some of the bowel contents of one person into another to substantially alter that person's bacterial population has assumed a level of credibility within medical circles (more on this in Chapter 7).

What remains an established fact, however, is that the odour of our bowel products, however putrid, really doesn't matter much at all. Over the years, many of my patients have complained to me about the intensely offensive odour of their own gas (or that of their partner); I have never yet been able to associate a single instance of this particular presenting complaint with any specific illness.

It is true that certain diseases are associated with particularly smelly bowel output – including mal-absorption syndromes such as lactose intolerance or fat malabsorption, and conditions that result in bleeding into the intestinal tract – but people with these diseases invariably complain of the symptoms of the underlying disease first and foremost. For these people, other symptoms predominate and the foul odour is secondary. For those whose complaint primarily focuses on the smell of their output, my experience has been that there is rarely if ever anything about which to be concerned.

Is it supposed to float?

As for buoyancy, here is the ultimate expression of an individual's conceit at the superiority of their own particular produce. Somewhere, sometime, someone noted with awe and pride that their stool was formed and floating, defiantly refusing to disappear discreetly down the S-bend, insisting on being noticed and admired in all its perfection of contour and colour. And when this was repeated on more than one occasion – and since such a well-formed stool was likely to have been complete, resulting in a comfortably empty feeling – its satisfied creator will have concluded that it was the floating that mattered most.

It seems almost certain that this was a man. Men often take close note of their bowel actions – probably looking out for that perfectly formed example of the species. Occasionally they will produce one in a public toilet and not even attempt to flush it away, imbued with the belief that others should be given the opportunity to view and admire this outstanding specimen. Other bulky and unusually buoyant bowel products simply defy every effort to flush them away, steadfastly floating on until time and erosion reduce them to ordinariness.

At the risk of deflating the pride of those self-congratulatory individuals described above, the buoyancy of any individual stool will be determined simply by its density. Certain specimens entrap gas within them and so tend to float. Others include little entrapped gas and so tend to sink. As noted above – and as we discuss in detail throughout this book – what matters in a bowel action is that it should be prompt, effortless, brief and complete. Whatever you subsequently see or do not see floating in the toilet bowl is irrelevant.

By all means, pursue a diet that helps you to achieve a formed stool (as we discuss later, consistency itself is important) and encourages the four characteristics outlined above. But do not pursue a diet specifically in search of a floating stool (or a sinker, for that matter). It matters not one jot whether our output sinks or floats, twirls, bobbles or corkscrews, rotating clockwise or counter. The output of a bowel action that is prompt, effortless, brief and complete is a good thing, whatever it subsequently does upon striking water.

Having cleared that up, let's get to know how the bowel actually works.

2

How the bowel works

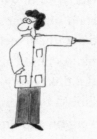

Our first step towards understanding how the bowel works is to understand the basic anatomy of a bowel action.

Anatomy of a bowel action

As Figure 1 illustrates, the small intestine starts where the stomach ends, and continues until the large intestine begins at the terminal ileum. (Note, in medical terminology, the terms *intestine* and *bowel* are interchangeable, so that small intestine is also known as the small bowel, and the large intestine also as the large bowel. However, throughout this book, for the sake of simplicity, we use the terms 'small intestine' and 'large intestine', the latter of which is synonymous with the everyday term 'bowel'.)

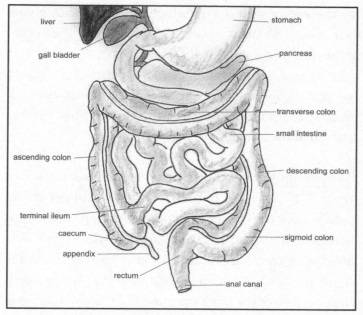

FIGURE 1. THE GASTROINTESTINAL TRACT

The large intestine comprises (in order) the colon, the rectum and the anus (also called the anal canal). The colon comprises (in order) the caecum (pronounced SEE-kum), the ascending colon, the transverse colon, the descending colon and the sigmoid colon.

The contents of the large intestine is called faeces (pronounced FEE-seas). The faeces that we pass out during a bowel action is referred to as a stool. The gas that we pass out is called flatus (pronounced FLAY-tus). What we eat generally takes about 24 hours to be expelled out the other end, but the pace of this journey varies at different stages. A comprehensive discussion of the entire process by which the food that enters our mouth comes to exit our body via the anal canal is beyond the scope of this brief book, so we'll start somewhere in the middle of that journey. Suffice it to say that the food we consume has already been chewed, swallowed, moistened and churned by the time it enters our small intestine.

The passage of food through our small intestine is very rapid. It is propelled by a series of powerful peristaltic (wave-like) muscle contractions through the entire length of the small intestine – during which time it is also being digested and its nutrients absorbed – and is dumped (now mostly in liquid form) into the caecum, the first part of the large intestine. The time it takes our food to get from our mouth to our colon is relatively short: three hours or less after a meal, virtually all of the food eaten at that meal has already entered the colon. At this point, however, things slow down considerably.

Our colon is a much more relaxed organ than the small intestine, happy for its contents to be stored for hours or even longer, until muscle contractions of generally only mild to moderate strength arise and move these contents (now called faeces) along its length. Propulsion through the colon occurs as a result of muscle-contraction waves referred to as 'mass movements'. These are provoked by a range of factors, which we'll look at in a moment. They occur with variable frequency and variable intensity among the human population. In some people these contraction waves are able to propel the entire contents of the bowel from caecum to rectum and out of the anus in one sitting, while in others they're often unable to nudge the faeces even a few centimetres.

Overall, however, a mass movement tends to propel faeces part but not all of the way around the large intestine. So the food you ate three hours ago for lunch might now be sitting in your caecum, a mass movement having moved what had previously been in your caecum (perhaps from breakfast this morning) around to your transverse colon or beyond. The next mass movement you experience will serve to propel your lunch from caecum to transverse colon and your breakfast from transverse colon down into your rectum, where it will demand to be expelled.

Colonic transit time

The time it takes for faeces to be moved through the entire large intestine – from when it first enters the caecum to when it is expelled through the anus in the course of a bowel action – is referred to as the *colonic transit time*.

As noted above, while the transit of food through the small intestine is predictably brisk, colonic transit time is generally slow. Any variation in how frequently different people open their bowels is thus much more likely to reflect variation in colonic transit time than differences in the speed of passage through the small intestine.

In other words, the time it takes the food we eat to be expelled from our bowels is primarily influenced by the colonic transit time and much less so by the generally fast and predictable transit through stomach and small intestine.

Numerous factors provoke the mass movements that propel faeces around the large intestine and so determine colonic transit time. These include the entry of food into the stomach upon eating (the so-called gastro-colic reflex); the entry of digested food from the small intestine into the caecum; specific chemicals in foods that stimulate these muscle contractions; physical exercise; and the simple act of getting up and out of bed. In many people, these factors aggregate each morning (getting up, eating breakfast, drinking a hot cup of coffee), which explains the most common human pattern of a daily bowel action in the morning.

Other factors that commonly influence our colonic transit time include what we eat (fruit, vegetables, caffeine, spicy foods and alcoholic drinks commonly speed things up); how much we eat (small-volume weight-loss diets often aggravate constipation); how much we exercise (a brisk walk can often provoke a strong urge); medications we are taking (a short list of commonly used medications that can cause trouble in either direction is provided in Chapter 6); and emotional stress, which tends to make whichever tendency we have – whether towards constipation or urgency – more marked.

But perhaps the most important factor influencing colonic transit time in humans is totally beyond our control – our sex. As it turns out, men and women have, on average, very different colonic transit times and, as a consequence, very different bowel habits and clinical presentations.

Mars and Venus in the bathroom

In a simple but compelling study performed at the University of Minnesota more than 30 years ago, the bowel habits of healthy adult men and women were compared. During the study, all the participants consumed identical amounts and types of food and drink, and the frequency of their bowel actions, the total weight of stool produced and even the volume of flatus expelled were measured. The study found that, on average, the men opened their bowels more often and produced a greater weight of stool and a greater volume of flatus than did the women.

When I describe the findings of this study to my patients, it rarely comes as a surprise to them. The majority of heterosexual couples have already made the same observations – he is fast and fruity; she is slow and sluggish. He gets up in the morning, puts his feet on the ground and heads straight to the bathroom; she gets up in the morning, puts her feet on the ground and asks herself, 'What am I going to have to eat and drink and do today to get my bowels to work?'

This is not to say that every man experiences swift colonic transit or that every woman experiences the reverse. Not at all. But it is simply inescapable that, as a general rule, men and women differ considerably in the workings of their bowels and in the sorts of bowel-related clinical problems they experience. (This difference is apparent from a very early age. As a venerable professor of paediatrics once told me during my medical-school years, boys are, as a general rule, 'good bowel athletes'.) All of this can be explained by the simple fact that women have consistently longer colonic transit times than men; unequivocally, on average, it takes longer for faeces to pass from caecum to rectum in women than it does in men.

Given the multitude of factors speeding up or slowing down colonic transit on an almost minute-by-minute basis, it should come as no surprise how greatly colonic transit time varies from day to day and from individual to individual. From the perspective of this book, then, it is the function of the large intestine that is most likely to vary between individuals, and which therefore clearly matters most in determining the nature of our bowel habits.

So what does the large intestine actually do?

Thanks to the hardworking small intestine, virtually all of the truly important absorption and nutritional activity of the intestines has well and truly been completed by the time the food we've swallowed reaches the large intestine. The large intestine produces no essential enzymes, secretes no vital hormones and absorbs no essential nutrients. It does absorb water and salt and some protein. But people can – and do – live absolutely normal lives from a dietary and nutritional perspective having had their entire large intestine surgically removed. So what's the point of it all?

In reality, the large intestine does little more than dry out faeces and coordinate its exit from the body at times that suit. The actions of the large intestine can, therefore, quite accurately be described as being of primarily social importance. It is all the more remarkable, then, that so much grief affecting so many people can be sheeted home to the fickle workings of this otherwise unimportant storage and expulsion organ.

The mechanics of defecation

So now we know what makes faeces move around the colon to the rectum. However, the last bit – the act of defecation, or emptying our bowels – represents an even more complex event, characterised by a mixture of intrinsic physiological factors and highly variable behavioural influences.

Ideally, a normally occurring mass movement will propel faeces through the colon and down into the rectum, where the rise in pressure inside the rectum will provoke an urge – a sense of the need to evacuate the rectum. The intensity of this urge will be determined by how great that rise in pressure is (what volume of faeces arrives in the rectum) and how quickly that rise in pressure occurs (how fast the faeces enters the rectum).

Imagine a situation such as a bout of gastroenteritis, or the effects of bowel preparation before a colonoscopy. In each case a large volume of fluid faeces enters a completely empty rectum at high speed. The rise in pressure is both great and rapid, and the accompanying urge is strong, even difficult to resist.

On the other hand, imagine someone who has been constipated for many years, and whose rectum is already distended by hard and dry faeces. A weak colonic contraction that propels additional faeces only slowly into the rectum might produce only a small and slow rise in pressure within the rectum, and so provoke a barely perceptible urge to evacuate.

To make things even more complicated, we also need to take into consideration the circumstances under which these changes in rectal pressure are taking place. Let's take a more usual situation here – a standard colonic contraction occurring in an 'average' large intestine, producing a good, strong urge but at a time and place when that person is unable to readily get to a bathroom. Maybe she is in a work meeting, in the car or at some distance from a clean and private facility. Whatever the reason, let's assume that she is not in a position to drop whatever she's doing and head off to the bathroom.

Luckily, most adult human beings are able to hold on in the presence of an urge of normal strength. This is because the rectum has the capacity to 'receptively relax'. While the entire small intestine and colon up to the rectum are programmed only to contract – and to keep on contracting – when distended by content, the rectum is able to distend and relax if need be. This allows the pressure within the rectum to be reduced, and the sense of needing to evacuate to ease, at least for a while.

Nearly everyone on the planet will have regularly taken advantage of this extremely useful ability of a normal, healthy rectum – to relax rather than contract – as a way of allowing them to delay having to visit a bathroom when it was not possible (or convenient) to do so. Of course, with successive mass movements and progressive distension of the rectum by faeces, the pressure increase will ultimately become sufficiently persuasive as to make a trip to the bathroom essential – and a great relief.

So, in the face of a strong urge occurring at a socially appropriate moment, we head to the bathroom, sit on the toilet and 'bear down' – an act that serves to relax our pelvic floor and our external anal sphincter muscle (Figure 2). This allows our anal canal to open

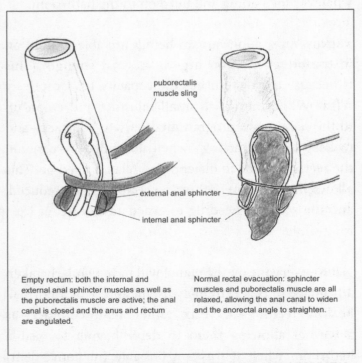

puborectalis muscle sling

external anal sphincter

internal anal sphincter

Empty rectum: both the internal and external anal sphincter muscles as well as the puborectalis muscle are active; the anal canal is closed and the anus and rectum are angulated.

Normal rectal evacuation: sphincter muscles and puborectalis muscle are all relaxed, allowing the anal canal to widen and the anorectal angle to straighten.

FIGURE 2. CHANGES IN ANAL SPHINCTER TONE AND ANORECTAL ANGLE AT REST AND DURING NORMAL RECTAL EVACUATION

and the angle between the rectum and the anal canal to straighten. In combination, this creates a favourable outlet for the passage of faeces (which is referred to as a 'stool' once it is at the point of exit). The act of bearing down also results in the rectum descending lower into the pelvis; this appears to stimulate a colonic and rectal contraction wave, which initiates propulsion of the stool.

The combined effects of a rectum distended by faeces, a colonic and rectal contraction wave and a wide-open, straight anorectal outlet (rectum and anal canal) provides the optimal circumstances for a stool to be expelled. Out comes the stool and the job is done. Hopefully, we are left feeling comfortably empty.

Without doubt, the natural state for the rectum is to be empty. The rectum is not meant to be a place for the prolonged storage of stool, but rather a place to receive and sense the arrival of faeces, holding things up until a strong urge has built and we have found an appropriate location to allow it to pass.

A quick note about anal disorders

Although it is beyond the scope of this book to describe the whole gamut of diseases that can affect the bowel, this is an opportune moment to point out that there are a few common and important causes of difficulty with rectal evacuation for which medical attention – careful clinical assessment and treatment – is required. Such correction often results in complete and lasting relief of symptoms.

Perhaps the most common condition that causes problems with rectal emptying is an anal fissure – a split or tear in the anal lining, just at the junction between inside and outside. Typically, such a fissure results in intense pain with the passage of a stool, and sometimes the appearance of bright-red blood on the toilet paper. Often, there is also a prolonged aching or throbbing pain around the anus that can last for minutes or even hours after a bowel action. All of these symptoms tend to be much worse when the stool that has been passed is large and hard.

Anal fissures are almost always associated with continuous spasm of the internal anal sphincter muscle, which is not under our voluntary control. For this reason, almost all of the effective treatments for anal fissures involve efforts to reduce this spasm – sphincter-relaxing creams, injections into the sphincter of the paralysing agent botox, or surgical cutting of the sphincter.

Where there is spasm of the internal anal sphincter and pain associated with defecation, rectal emptying can never be prompt or effortless, and can rarely be quick or complete. So whenever there is an anal fissure present, correcting the internal anal sphincter spasms and healing the fissure are the first and most important steps in restoring normal rectal emptying.

Another potential cause of difficulty with rectal evacuation is narrowing or stricture of the anal canal. This is not especially common, but can be a consequence of previous anal surgery (such as a haemorrhoidectomy) or part of the inflammatory condition known as Crohn's disease.

The anal canal can also be the site of malignant lesions or ulcers (anal cancer), which are also often painful and frequently cause bleeding. These can readily be detected by a doctor on the basis of simple inspection and internal digital examination.

Overall, these conditions form only a minority of cases in my own practice – but no progress can ever be made and much time can be wasted until they have been diagnosed and properly treated. Your family doctor is the person best placed to exclude these various diagnoses or to recommend the most appropriate course of action should one be present.

3

Getting the process started: how do we know when it's time to go?

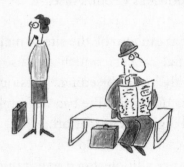

Since we've already observed that every truly successful bowel action is associated with prompt initiation, it's important to understand exactly what enables satisfactory commencement.

From a practical perspective, it's the strength and the quality of the urge to defecate that most closely correlates with the speed and ease of doing so. Entering the bathroom with a good, strong urge is a reliable harbinger of prompt and effortless rectal emptying. Put simply, a good bowel action depends more on the presence of a strong and true urge to empty the rectum than on any other single thing.

Conversely, any trip to the bathroom undertaken in the presence of only a weak or indifferent urge reliably forecasts delayed or difficult initiation of defecation, and so heralds the need to strain to get things going. A weak urge is also likely to result in prolonged and incomplete defecation, due to the sheer lack of propulsive force. Discomfort, frustration, demoralisation and even depression can and do follow.

Therefore, for the process of defecation to get going promptly and effortlessly, and for rectal emptying to be brief and complete – those four important characteristics of a satisfactory bowel action – the urge that takes us to the bathroom must be strong and true. This is the single most important rule of good bowel function, so it deserves the title of Golden Rule Number One. (When speaking to my patients, I often refer to it as 'The Eleventh Commandment'.)

Golden Rule Number One
Never attempt to empty your bowel until the urge to do so is strong and true.

Our ability to allow an unequivocally strong urge to develop before visiting the bathroom really is the absolute crux of having a good bowel action, and of achieving a good bowel habit. Make no mistake: urge is king.

What could possibly go wrong?

For many people, getting to a bathroom to empty their bowels at the right time is a straightforward matter about which not a moment's thought need ever be given. These people would find it hard to imagine that a bowel action could be anything other than simple, natural and utterly effortless. But there are a number of ways in which – and very many people for whom – it is all too easy to arrive at the bathroom without a truly 'irresistible' urge.

Some people – people who are perfectly capable of distinguishing a strong urge from a weak one – choose to go to the bathroom before the arrival of an urge of suitable quality out of habit or misguided personal preference. Others simply never achieve an urge of adequate strength – at least not without artificial assistance. And some misinterpret signals from their bowel or elsewhere and head to the bathroom in the false belief that a bowel action is imminent.

If you are one of those plagued by an inability to initiate rectal evacuation promptly and effortlessly, I hope you will find an explanation and some assistance here.

Pre-emptive or premature defecation: a case of bad timing

Logically, all of us should only ever go to the bathroom when we have the need to do so right away. In this scenario, we would recognise that critical sensation, stop what we were doing, head to the bathroom, complete the task with a minimum of fuss and effort and leave the bathroom to resume whatever we were previously doing.

But almost every human being on the planet has, at one time or another, elected to go to the bathroom not out of pressing necessity but out of perceived convenience. 'If I go now, before I leave home, I won't have to worry about it later.' Some people make a habit out of this practice, sitting on the toilet for tactical reasons more often than they do in a truly timely fashion. I refer to this habit as *pre-emptive defecation* – obliging one's bowel to work when there is essentially no natural urge to do so.

Others consider the timing of their trips to the bathroom a matter of personal ritual. 'I always go right after breakfast.' This is often based on the person's experience that their bowel generally does work in the mornings, but by entering the bathroom in advance of the arrival of an appropriately strong urge – often with newspaper or mobile device in hand – they are, in effect, 'sitting on the platform, waiting for the train to arrive'. I refer to this pattern as *premature defecation* – anticipating the working of one's bowel when the appropriately strong urge is still some way off.

These two varieties of anticipation are all well and good as they relate to our bladders – in fact, human beings often visit the bathroom to empty their bladders out of convenience, well before they are 'busting to go'. We do this for very good reasons and without doing ourselves any disservice at all. Before going in to see a movie, before heading in to a meeting, before starting a long car trip or – in my case – before beginning a long operation, we regularly empty our bladders to avoid the inconvenience of having to interrupt our upcoming activity. But the same logic should never be applied to our bowels, for a couple of very good reasons.

First, unlike the rectum, which is a rather weak muscular structure, the bladder is a powerful one that can readily push out even tiny amounts of urine when requested to do so. Second, also unlike the rectum, the bladder cannot receptively relax once it is full: once it reaches a certain degree of fullness, we simply cannot ignore the need for our bladder to be emptied. So a full bladder, unlike a full rectum, cannot be ignored or put off. The bowel and the bladder are thus radically different parts of the body, and we should not for one minute imagine that we can empty our bowels at any convenient time in the same way as we regularly do with our bladders. And so back to the bowel. In 'textbook' cases of pre-emptive or premature defecation, the person affected is in fact perfectly able to achieve a pressing urge to evacuate their bowel and therefore to permit prompt and effortless initiation of evacuation. It is their decision to sit on the toilet in advance of the arrival of such an urge that accounts for the delay in initiation and the need for straining. This problem is generally, therefore, a matter of faulty toileting behaviour – a case of bad timing.

It is also very common for pre-emptive and premature defecators to make matters worse by entering the bathroom with reading material in hand – newspapers, books, magazines, laptops, tablets, mobile phones. This is an important cause of people spending too much time sitting on the toilet, and leads us to Golden Rule Number Two.

Golden Rule Number Two
Never, ever take any distracting influences
– newspapers, books, magazines, mobile devices –
with you to the bathroom.

Without doubt, excessive time spent sitting on the toilet is a significant contributor to haemorrhoidal congestion and associated symptoms of bleeding and protrusion. And distractions such as reading material and mobile devices actually disguise the fact that you should not really be sitting there at all, and serve as a kind of reward for poor toileting behaviour.

The reality is that the very reason people choose to take such distractions with them to the bathroom is precisely because they know they are likely to be spending a lot of time in there. It's a case of, 'Rather than waiting for the arrival of a strong urge before going to the bathroom, why not go early, read the paper and see what happens?' It's little wonder that evacuation proves unsatisfactory when people elect to go to the bathroom as much to catch up on the news as to empty their bowels.

So, if you are a person who suffers from an inability to initiate rectal evacuation promptly and effortlessly, then, rather than using your bathroom as a library or a home office, you must consciously avoid ever taking any distracting influences – any at all – with you when you visit the bathroom. That way, if you find yourself sitting there waiting for things to get started, you will be totally focused on the truth of the matter: that you have not waited until the urge was strong enough, that this is why you have been unable to achieve prompt and effortless initiation of rectal emptying, and that you should not be sitting there at all.

Essentially, the solution to the problem of arriving at the bathroom before the urge to evacuate is appropriately strong is the application of Golden Rule Number One. The remedy for both pre-emptive and premature defecators is to consciously delay attempting defecation until the urge to do so is *irresistible*. I contend that every bathroom door on the planet should have a sign on the outside that reads: 'Unless you are truly busting to open your bowel this instant, back off!'

This issue is not just about wasted time – although pre-emptive and premature defecators do often spend an inordinate amount of time in the bathroom, which can be deeply frustrating. It is also about the fact that the (self-caused) need to strain to get things started can have consequences – haemorrhoids that bleed and/ or protrude, pelvic-floor muscular discomfort and pain – that often give rise to the need to seek medical assistance.

So, for people who have normal or even rapid colonic transit – as is often the case in men – all that is generally needed to address these complaints is to correct this common behavioural problem by delaying defecation until the urge to go is strong. But, alas, these habits can be hard to eradicate.

Pre-emptive defecators often dread having to open their bowels at work or in a public place – or, for that matter, anywhere at all on the planet other than at home in the privacy of their own bathroom. Often this is because they believe that, since their pre-emptive efforts at home take them such a long time to initiate and complete, any other attempt to evacuate will take a similarly long time. They have lost confidence in their innate ability to achieve prompt initiation of defecation, and so their pattern of pre-emptive visits becomes ever more entrenched.

In truth, if they would only get out of the habit of pre-emptively visiting the bathroom and instead adopt the much more natural process of consciously awaiting the arrival of a powerful urge, they would appreciate the vastly shorter amount of time needed in the bathroom and an altogether more satisfying toileting experience.

Premature defecators are also very attached to the privacy and solitude of their own bathroom. For them, their bathroom has become a refuge from the outside world. They enjoy the time it gives them to read or to check their emails. I have had many patients who have come to appreciate that their toileting behaviours are the root cause of their difficulties with initiation of defecation, or the principal explanation for their haemorrhoids or their pelvic-floor discomfort. But when push comes to shove, they simply will not stop what they have been doing for many years.

However, when the time and effort spent 'sitting on the platform, waiting for the train to arrive' takes its toll in the form of discomfort, haemorrhoids and plain frustration, the solution becomes much more acceptable. Premature defecators need to read that imaginary sign on the outside of their bathroom door, and delay their arrival onto the platform until the conductor yells: 'All aboard!'

In summary, for people with normal colonic transit time, rectal evacuation can and should be prompt and effortless every time. All it takes is adherence to the notion of delaying trips to the bathroom until the urge is strong, combined with the discipline of never taking any distracting reading material or electronic devices to the bathroom.

Slow-colonic-transit constipation: where the urge to go is weak or absent

There are many people who never readily experience that truly irresistible urge to empty their bowels. As already discussed, the ability of human beings to perceive the urge to evacuate depends upon sufficient faeces entering an empty rectum at sufficient speed to generate a quick and substantial rise in pressure within the rectum.

Contrast the sensation generated by the rapid arrival of voluminous bowel content under the influence of bowel preparation for a colonoscopy (which can result in an overwhelmingly strong urge that threatens continence) with the sensation associated with a weak contraction wave in a person with slow-colonic-transit constipation whose rectum is already occupied by faeces built up over preceding hours or even days. This latter sensation might, at best, evince a vague inkling to go.

The reality is that slow-colonic-transit constipation is common. It affects, to some degree, almost half of the adult female population of the planet. While it can be mild and intermittent in many women, it is not infrequently a significant impediment to normal quality of life. Infrequent and weak urges to evacuate, prominent abdominal bloating, straining to evacuate and ever-increasing dependence on laxatives are its characteristic symptoms. Onset may be in childhood, but it is often first noticed in the mid-teens, when travelling, dieting and other seemingly minor life changes can aggravate symptoms. Pregnancy, childbirth or undergoing surgical procedures might precipitate a substantial exacerbation.

In this group, failure to achieve a satisfactory urge is inherent in the underlying sluggish colonic transit. As a result, sufferers get into the habit of visiting the bathroom when the urge to go is as close to strong as they are likely to experience. They soon appreciate that missing that singular opportunity to go is likely to mean that, when another urge – any urge at all – next arises, the prospect of being able to go will only have diminished further. Their bowel contents by that time will have become even harder and drier. These women – and the majority of this group are women – therefore come to appreciate the importance of recognising and responding to that urge, even though it is rarely pressing.

They also appreciate that the circumstances need to be right for evacuation to occur – the right sort of bathroom with the right degree of privacy. All the 'stars' need to be in alignment if they are going to achieve satisfactory evacuation in response to the urge that has arisen. I am sure that anyone reading this who suffers from slow colonic transit will recognise this description as the sort of conundrum they regularly face.

This is a tough situation for the sufferer, especially as the solution runs contrary to widely held but totally misguided medical and public sentiment. The solution to an inability to experience a truly pressing urge in those with slow colonic transit rests with creating such an urge by artificial means – in short, the solution here requires the use of laxatives.

Sadly, 'laxative' is still a dirty word all over the world. But without a shadow of doubt, the appropriate use of appropriate laxatives represents the very best and the most suitable way to go in this situation. Correct use of laxatives enables the sufferer to generate an urge to evacuate of sufficient strength to permit satisfactory rectal evacuation. I spend more time discussing laxatives in Chapter 5.

Speculative defecation: a false alarm

The process of opening one's bowel involves a complex interplay of physical, physiological and behavioural factors. A typical and successful bowel action involves a physical sensation (the urge to go) in response to a genuine physiological event (rising pressure within the rectum), which then prompts a behavioural response (the decision to go to the bathroom and attempt rectal evacuation).

A significant subgroup of people who suffer from difficulty with the initiation and completion of defecation do so because the physical sensation in response to which they elect to go to the bathroom is not associated with a genuine physiological need to go. They think they need to go but the sensation to which they are responding falls well short of (or does not correspond at all to) the sort of physiological event necessary to permit prompt and effortless initiation of defecation.

In these cases, the physical sensation they experience is misinterpreted as a real urge. But because the physical sensation turns out to be a false alarm and because the urge turns out to be insufficient, these people reach the bathroom with an inadequate urge. As a consequence, initiation is delayed and straining is required to effect any sort of evacuation at all. Frustration is profound, since these individuals are quite convinced that the need to be there is real.

In truth, sufferers in this situation have often lost their ability to discern between 'the real thing' and what are just false alarms. They think that the physical sensations they have should allow them to get their bowels to work. They are undoubtedly uncomfortable, but they are by no means 'busting to go'. They go to the bathroom in the hope that opening their bowels will rid them of their misleading and uncomfortable sensation. I describe this pattern of defecation as *speculative defecation* – going in response to a sensation that is not a true and pressing urge, hoping for (rather than confident of) success.

Speculative visits to the bathroom are inevitably unsatisfactory, since they occur in the absence of that all-important powerful urge. Consequently, initiation is delayed, straining is required and evacuation is rarely complete.

And matters can become even more complicated. Voluntary straining in an attempt to get rid of the annoying feeling of needing to go frequently has the unwanted

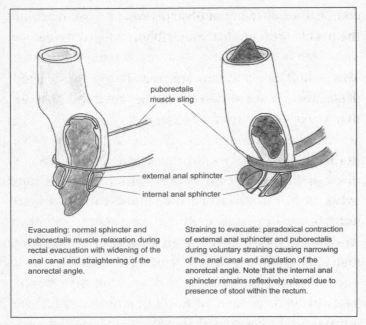

puborectalis
muscle sling

external anal sphincter

internal anal sphincter

Evacuating: normal sphincter and puborectalis muscle relaxation during rectal evacuation with widening of the anal canal and straightening of the anorectal angle.

Straining to evacuate: paradoxical contraction of external anal sphincter and puborectalis during voluntary straining causing narrowing of the anal canal and angulation of the anoretcal angle. Note that the internal anal sphincter remains reflexively relaxed due to presence of stool within the rectum.

FIGURE 3. PARADOXICAL EXTERNAL AND SPHINCTER
CONTRACTION CAUSED BY VOLUNTARY STRAINING

effect of causing contraction of the pelvic floor and anal sphincter, thereby narrowing and angulating the anorectal outlet. This is the opposite of the wide-open, straight anorectal outlet that is supposed to arise when we bear down to empty our bowels (Figure 3).

Voluntary straining can therefore have the paradoxical effect of narrowing the anorectal outlet at the precise time that the speculative defecator wants it to be at its widest and straightest. In addition to an inadequate urge, then, they must cope with what is, in effect, an obstructed anorectal outlet. Sufferers characteristically complain of a feeling of obstruction, and can describe the passage of flattened, even ribbon-shaped, faeces.

This situation is often referred to as 'obstructed defecation'. These sufferers can be utterly convinced that they have a fixed mechanical obstruction, and are often incredulous when, after a thorough physical examination including the passage of a broad speculum through the anus, they are told that no such obstruction exists. In truth, of course, they do have an obstruction, but it is only present when they engage in voluntary straining and it is therefore an obstruction entirely of their own making, albeit quite unintended.

Speculative defecation is, not surprisingly, an utterly infuriating affliction, and one that has a tendency to deteriorate over time. This is because it is common for human beings to respond to having taken a long time to effect rectal evacuation by actually allowing themselves even more time to go. Rather than delaying their visits to the bathroom until the arrival of a genuinely pressing urge, they are fearful about how much time they will need to get things out and so opt to visit the bathroom earlier and earlier, in response to progressively more vague physical sensations.

Not surprisingly, as the sensations to which they respond move further and further away from that ideal and irresistible urge that would have given them a fighting chance of initiating a bowel action promptly, and as their visits to the bathroom become more and more speculative, they experience more and more difficulty in initiating defecation. And, as their voluntary straining increases, paradoxically narrowing their anorectal outlet and causing obstruction at this critical time, they descend into a demoralising spiral of ever more speculative timing, weaker urges and more severe anorectal outlet narrowing.

So how does this all start? How does someone who once experienced irresistible urges and effected perfectly satisfactory bowel actions get to the point of sitting on the toilet in a progressively more speculative manner, utterly convinced that they should be trying to go but ever more anxious that evacuation will not start promptly, and that it will be accompanied by the need for straining and the unshakable sense of an obstructed outlet?

There are two pathways to this unhappy endpoint, and most sufferers have gone down both pathways to varying degrees. One is the slow-colonic-transit pathway – having inherently weak urges to open one's bowel is a common starting point for speculative defecation. The other is the behavioural pathway – this involves bad timing and normal physical sensations being misinterpreted. The solution to the problem of speculative defecation therefore requires a dual approach, in which colonic transit time is sped up by using laxatives and behaviour is modified by means of a simple approach I refer to as *The Three Ds* (see below). Laxatives will be especially important in people with unambiguous slow-colonic-transit constipation, but even in those with apparently normal colonic transit, laxative therapy can prove useful by provoking especially speedy colonic transit and, as a result, truly powerful urges. By assisting the sufferer to experience a genuinely irresistible urge – sometimes for the first time in many months or even years – laxatives can enable them to distinguish this correct, strong urge from weaker, more speculative urges.

The Three Ds

The Three Ds refers to a simple behavioural approach to correct the faulty toileting behaviour associated with speculative defecation. It works as follows.

Defer Speculative defecators must make a conscious decision to defer visiting the bathroom until the urge to go is strong and true, thus adhering to that first and most important Golden Rule for a satisfying bowel action and a satisfactory bowel habit. This is all about that imaginary sign on the outside of the bathroom door that reads: 'Unless you are truly busting to open your bowel this instant, back off!'

Desist Notwithstanding their (misjudged) feeling of wanting to go, speculative defecators find that rectal evacuation simply will not get going either promptly or effortlessly. But once someone has made the decision to set aside time to visit the bathroom, hoping to relieve their discomfort by effecting some degree of rectal emptying, they are likely to want to justify that decision regardless of their misjudgement. In other words, even though rectal emptying does not commence, a speculative defecator will stay on the toilet, sit and strain in an attempt to go. This serves only to aggravate their problems and exacerbate their pelvic-floor discomfort. They seek to reward their bad timing by insisting on getting some result, however small, and at whatever cost in terms of effort, discomfort and frustration.

Rather than sit and strain, speculative defecators must desist – they need to acknowledge that rectal evacuation has not commenced promptly and that this is because they have entered the bathroom in the absence of an appropriately strong urge. As such, they need to get up and leave the bathroom immediately. They must not reward the bad timing that got them into this trouble in the first place.

There should, then, be another sign on the inside of every bathroom door on the planet that reads: 'If you have been here for 30 seconds and nothing has happened, you must have got it wrong. Do not sit and strain – get up and leave this instant!'

Distinguish The essential issue for speculative defecators is their inability to distinguish between real urges and false alarms. By deferring and desisting, they will hopefully spend ever less time and exert ever less effort in the process of getting their bowels to work. Ultimately, however, their task is to learn all over again how to distinguish those bodily sensations that will reliably lead to prompt and effortless initiation of defecation from those that will result only in frustrating delay and difficulty. Developing this ability to distinguish between real and false signals is the essence of correcting speculative defecation and its associated problems of straining, haemorrhoids and pelvic-floor pain.

Opportunistic defecation: while I'm here, I might as well

A quite different problem is more often associated with overactive bowels, where colonic transit is, if anything, too brisk. As a consequence, the colon transmits soft faeces around to the rectum steadily and consistently during the day. For some individuals with this sort of colonic overactivity, normally occurring visits to the toilet to empty their bladders are, at the last minute, accompanied by an unanticipated urge to use their bowels.

For these people, the presence of some soft faeces in the rectum – insufficient on its own to generate an urge to open their bowels – becomes apparent only once urination commences. This is possibly because relaxation of the urinary sphincter (to allow the passage of urine) also involves relaxation and lowering of the pelvic floor. This appears to provoke a left-sided colonic contraction, which might deliver just enough additional faeces into the rectum to create a sensation of the need for it to be emptied.

Before entering the bathroom, this person did not anticipate the need to open their bowel. Once there, however, they recognise the sensation of rectal filling and, since they are in the vicinity, take the opportunity to relieve themselves of it, conveniently 'killing two birds with one stone'. That is why I refer to this phenomenon as *opportunistic defecation* – going when a bowel action was not the initial purpose of the visit but because the opportunity (rather than the need) arose and so was duly obliged.

This sensation is a little more likely to be noticed by women, who have of course sat down to empty their bladders. But men, too, can find that a visit they imagined would be over in a matter of seconds needs to be redirected and extended. Regardless of the sex of the sufferer, this last-minute perceived need to effect rectal evacuation is inconvenient. Moreover, this kind of urge to empty the rectum is never truly full-blooded and so is, as already discussed, likely to be associated with incomplete and unsatisfactory evacuation. Accordingly, opportunistic defecators find this entire experience unsatisfactory – a sub-optimal urge and softer-than-ideal stool consistency combine to result in incomplete emptying of soft, sticky faeces.

Opportunistic defecators complain of not feeling empty and of the need to use a lot of toilet paper to clean up; they often leave the bathroom feeling thoroughly frustrated at the discomfort associated with their failure to fully empty, and the unexpected time taken for what they originally imagined would be a brief visit. Likewise, they are annoyed at the sheer inconvenience associated with the lengthy and messy process of wiping up.

Since we are able to empty our bladders even when they are only partly filled with urine, it is absolutely normal for human beings to empty their bladders whenever they sit down to have a bowel action. But the reverse is not the case: since our bowels are only meant to work when the urge to do so is strong and true, it is not usual – and definitely not intended – that our bowels should work whenever we go to pass urine. If opportunistic defecation is a recurring problem for you, it can and should be corrected.

The solution, in this case, is to slow down your colonic transit time, in order to allow stool consistency to become firmer. As I elaborate in Chapter 4, the ideal consistency of a human stool is solid and well formed, not soft and sloppy. For opportunistic defecators, the root cause of their problem is fast-moving and soft faeces; by slowing down their colonic transit time and allowing stool consistency to become more solid, they are generally able to return to a more usual pattern of mass movements that allows them to experience strong urges to empty their bowels quite independent of their bathroom visits for urination.

The importance of solid stool consistency and the ways to achieve the ideal stool is covered in detail in Chapter 4.

4

Completing the process: the importance of being empty

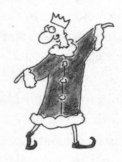

An empty bowel is a happy bowel.

There is no doubt in my mind that the natural state for the entire intestine is to be empty. The small intestine is such a vigorous propellant that any individual segment of it is rarely full for more than a few seconds. The large intestine, on the other hand, is regularly cast in the role of storage organ. But it, too, is only ever truly happy when it has also propelled its contents along and beyond, leaving itself decompressed, comfortable and able to rest and recover its natural elasticity, and thereby retain its inherent capacity to contract again when needed.

Let's consider this issue in terms of the large intestine's two main parts: the colon and the rectum.

The colon likes to be empty

If we were to take a simple X-ray of a human abdomen at any time of any day, we would most likely be able to see the presence of faeces – as well as gas – within the colon (and even the rectum). This, of course, is where faeces rightfully belongs. However, like the rest of the intestinal tract, the colon is a muscular tube that exists to propel its contents forwards, and it struggles when it cannot do so efficiently.

A normally functioning colon will contract and propel its contents forwards in response to numerous factors, as described in Chapter 2. But, like any elastic structure, if it is overstretched its muscular walls will become thinner and less powerful in their ability to contract and propel faeces along its length.

The colon of a person with inherently slow colonic transit is likely to propel faeces slowly and incompletely; sufferers of slow-colonic-transit constipation routinely describe their inability to completely empty their bowels. So it is these individuals – who already struggle to propel faeces effectively – who are most at risk of experiencing incomplete colonic emptying resulting in overstretching of the colonic wall and, hence, even less effective faecal propulsion.

Here, then, is a vicious circle: weak colonic propulsion favours incomplete colonic emptying, which favours overstretching of the colon, which in turn favours even weaker propulsion, and so on. This explains the natural tendency of constipation to progressively deteriorate over time. It also explains the absolute importance of achieving total colonic emptying when using laxatives to treat constipation. (This is explained in more detail in Chapter 5, which deals at length with laxative use.)

That lucky person who gets up every morning, puts his feet on the ground (it is more often a man than a woman) and heads straight to the bathroom to reliably enjoy a satisfactory bowel action does so precisely because, when he went to the bathroom to open his bowel the previous day, he left the bathroom completely empty. This is because a totally empty colon is able to rest and recover its inherent elasticity and contractility so that the following day it will respond again with appropriate vigour to the forces that naturally encourage it to contract and propel.

A completely empty colon is a sure recipe for the maintenance of muscular elasticity and contractility, helping to maintain forceful bowel contractions and complete bowel emptying. Conversely, an incompletely empty colon represents the first stage in a steady decline towards troublesome constipation.

The rectum likes to be empty

In the course of my clinical career I have spoken to literally thousands of individuals about the workings of their bowels. Almost everyone I have ever spoken to has been able to recall the sensation of having left the bathroom with a truly empty rectum – and to recall that experience with considerable affection. If they have been really lucky, this will have been a regular, perhaps daily experience. But even if it has only been an occasional or even an unequivocally rare event, the feeling that follows a bowel action that leaves the rectum totally empty is an unmistakably positive life experience.

When we achieve a completely empty rectum, we register three somewhat separate sensations. First, there is the immediate awareness that the rectum is completely empty – the rectum accurately senses the presence of even small amounts of residual stool and, equally accurately, reliably tells us when it is completely empty. Then there is the reassuring shutting tight of the anus – the feeling that the anus has sealed completely – created by the restoration of full contraction of the internal anal sphincter in response to the absence of any stool within the rectum. Third, there is the confirmatory absence of residual faeces when wiping up – on the very first wipe the toilet paper is clean, almost as if nothing has happened.

Without doubt, this is how we were intended to do business – and the satisfaction and pride experienced by human beings when they leave the bathroom with a completely empty rectum and a tightly shut anus is universal. Make no mistake: the objective of every bowel action is the complete emptying of the rectum.

An empty bowel is indeed a happy bowel.

As outlined in Chapter 3, straining to initiate a bowel action due to a weak, mistimed or misleading urge is an undeniably frustrating experience. But failure to completely empty the rectum when attempting to do so is every bit as infuriating. So what causes incomplete rectal emptying, and how can it be corrected? Before we answer this, there is an even more basic question to be considered.

What's wrong with not completely emptying the rectum?

Why is leaving the bathroom with an incompletely empty rectum such a problem?

Well, first and foremost, it is an undeniably unsatisfactory experience. As I have already said, the rectum is generally an accurate sensor of its own degree of emptiness, and when we do not empty it completely, we not only recognise that this is so, we recognise it as uncomfortable and annoying. Put simply, it feels 'wrong', and leaving the bathroom at that point requires us to consciously override an unshakable belief that we really should still be sitting down and waiting for more to happen.

So, even though the urge to evacuate has well and truly passed, the inescapable sensation of residual faeces within the rectum almost obliges us to try to get rid of that last bit. And we try to achieve this by straining. As we all know, straining can be uncomfortable and even tiring. Moreover, such voluntary straining is rarely completely effective, especially as it can, paradoxically, result in contraction of the pelvic floor muscles and narrowing of the external anal sphincter (see Figure 3 on page 46).

Over time, repeated and incompletely effective straining proves exhausting and frustrating. It also strains and even stretches the pelvic floor muscles, causing pelvic floor pain and weakness. So the need to strain to achieve complete rectal emptying is infuriating and draining, time-consuming and even painful. Clearly, it is something we do not want to have to do.

But there's more. If we leave the bathroom with an incompletely empty rectum, we are also prone to another adverse consequence: unconscious soiling or leakage of the retained stool.

There is a very important reflex affecting the rectum and anal sphincter muscles, which is known as the recto-anal inhibitory reflex. When it works as it should, this reflex means that as faeces descends into the lower rectum in anticipation of its imminent evacuation, the internal anal sphincter muscle reflexively relaxes, allowing the anus to adopt a more open pose for the bowel action that will soon follow.

The pelvic floor and the external anal sphincter are under our conscious control, so we can cause them to relax as we bear down. But the anal outlet can only be optimally open if, in addition, the internal anal sphincter also relaxes. Since we do not have conscious control over the internal anal sphincter, we rely on this recto-anal inhibitory reflex to ensure that the internal anal sphincter is also relaxed as the stool approaches the lower rectum, exactly when it needs to be.

Of course, if we fail to completely empty the rectum and instead leave the bathroom with even a small amount of retained faeces within the lower rectum, the internal anal sphincter remains reflexively relaxed in anticipation of the prospect of further rectal emptying. As a result, anal tone at rest remains low, permitting the faecal residue to leak out onto the perianal skin (the skin around the anus). This is especially likely to occur if that retained faeces is soft and if, after leaving the bathroom, we then engage in physical exertion – walking, housework, lifting and so on – which raises the pressure within the abdomen and literally squeezes the faecal residue out of the incompletely sealed anal canal.

Passive faecal soiling is an unhappy situation for everyone. The leakage is often entirely unconscious and can cause discomfort, irritation, itching and soreness once it has leaked onto the skin. Chafing and even bleeding can follow. It can also be smelly, and sufferers are often very self-conscious, anxious that others will have noticed. All in all, faecal soiling is a genuinely unpleasant event, and a very common reason patients are referred to see me.

What causes incomplete rectal emptying?

I think we can all now agree that incomplete rectal emptying is an unequivocally bad thing. But what accounts for it, and how can we correct it?

As I made clear in the previous chapter, the indisputable prerequisite for any truly satisfactory bowel action is to ensure that you reach the bathroom with a strong and true urge to evacuate. This, as already discussed, is Golden Rule Number One – the fundamental basis of every successful bowel action in recorded human history and a vital prerequisite for being able to leave the bathroom with a completely empty rectum. Without that irresistible urge, evacuation will not only be more difficult to initiate but will also be less likely to be complete.

So the first and most important cause of incomplete rectal emptying is exactly the same as the first and most important cause of difficulty with initiating rectal evacuation: failure to reach the bathroom with an appropriately forceful urge to do so. In this respect, people who engage in pre-emptive, premature or speculative defecation are all likely to experience difficulties with the completion of rectal evacuation, just as they can experience problems with its initiation. The recommendations provided in Chapter 3, which are designed to help people to achieve that strong and true urge to initiate evacuation, are therefore just as pertinent to those experiencing difficulty completing evacuation.

However, difficulty completing rectal evacuation can also be seen in people with seemingly strong urges to evacuate – and, indeed, with seemingly good colonic transit and even seemingly soft and free-moving bowel actions. Undoubtedly, then, urge is not the only factor that contributes to incomplete rectal emptying and subsequent post-defecation soiling. And this leads us to the third Golden Rule for happy and healthy rectal evacuation: the pursuit of a solid stool.

Golden Rule Number Three
The ideal consistency for a human stool is solid.

That's right. Notwithstanding the relentless emphasis in modern society on the health benefits of dietary fibre, the ideal consistency for a stool is, in fact, solid. By this I do not mean that the stool should be hard and pellet-like. Rather, it should have the shape and consistency (although definitely not the colour) of a peeled, unripe banana. The passage of precisely such a stool is likely to result in those three signs of an empty rectum – the sensation of rectal emptiness, the tight closure of the anal canal and the absence of faecal residue on the toilet paper.

Again, almost every person I have ever spoken to about their bowel habit has been able to recall – even if only from the distant past – the passage of such a 'big banana', as well as the satisfying, almost life-affirming, pleasure associated with its accomplishment. Without question, this is a good feeling; solid stool is very much what we are designed to produce. Alas, very few human beings manage to produce the perfect stool even just two days in a row, let alone consistently.

The importance of solid stool consistency for complete rectal emptying

As we all know, when stool consistency is too hard and dry – often as a result of slow colonic transit – initiating evacuation can be extremely difficult. But it is also true that when stool consistency is too soft, completing evacuation can be next to impossible.

Excessively soft stool consistency is a major cause of incomplete rectal emptying and thus of all the problems and unpleasant symptoms it causes. That our stool is soft suggests reasonably swift colonic transit, meaning that as long as we get the timing right we should be able to reach the bathroom with a good, strong urge that will at least enable us to initiate evacuation promptly and effortlessly. But the muscle-contraction wave that normally expels faeces in human beings is gentle and undulating rather than vigorous and muscular. So, once a stool is about halfway out, there really is little or no ongoing muscle contraction to assist in the completion of normal rectal evacuation.

Human beings rely, therefore, on the fact that when that contraction wave fades away, the part of the stool that is still inside the rectum remains mechanically attached to the part that is already out. In this manner, gravity and momentum assist the remainder of the stool to be expelled. If our stool consistency is too soft, the part that is already outside the rectum is likely to break off and fall into the toilet bowl, leaving some stool in and just outside the anus, as well as some more that is marooned higher up, inside the rectum.

In such a circumstance, we note three things. First, we do not feel as if we have finished the job (because we haven't). Second, the anus will not shut tight (because the residue of faeces left inside the rectum keeps the recto-anal inhibitory reflex activated, so keeping the internal anal sphincter relaxed). And third, we require a lot of wiping and many sheets of toilet paper to get ourselves clean (and even then we don't seem to be able to wipe up completely). This really is a time-consuming and entirely unsatisfactory experience, and it all results from having stool that is too soft.

Even if the first part of a stool is solid, many people find that stool consistency becomes progressively softer and less formed as the stool emerges. A single bowel action can start out quite solid but can then 'degenerate' as it emerges into a porridge-like or even pasty consistency. It is this soft and unformed component that is last to exit and therefore most likely to be left behind and, as a result, most likely to leak out on to the perianal skin after we have left the bathroom.

The pursuit of solid stool consistency is therefore absolutely critical if rectal evacuation is to be complete.

In combination with a strong urge to evacuate, it represents a vital part of the formula for a successful and satisfying bowel action. But how can we achieve it?

How to achieve solid stool consistency

If our stool consistency is too soft, how can it be rendered more solid? And how can this be achieved without going too far the other way, resulting in a stool that is too hard and dry and so results in constipation? There are essentially two ways we can make our stools firmer and more well formed. One is by dietary manipulation, and the other is through the use of medication. Many people reject out of hand the use of medication, believing that dietary manipulation is the more 'natural' approach. While I do not necessarily agree with this sentiment, let's at least start by considering how we can manipulate our diet to achieve that all-important 'big banana'.

Achieving solid stool consistency through diet

One view that is widely held is that certain foods tend to constipate us: white bread and meat are two commonly cited culprits. In reality, we are more likely to become constipated by eating nothing at all than we are by eating only white bread and meat.

Food is fuel not only for the generation of energy but very much also for the stimulation of our bowels. Recall from Chapter 2 that two of the factors that provoke the mass movements that propel faeces around our large intestine (and out through the rectum) are the entry of swallowed food into our stomach and the entry of digested food into our large intestine. No food in, no stool out. We are therefore much better advised to consider the effects of diet on stool consistency by looking at whether we are eating too much or too little of the foods that make our stools softer, rather than by focusing solely on foods that we think might be making us constipated.

There are many things that we eat and drink that undeniably speed up colonic transit, rendering our bowel actions faster-moving, more urgent and more liquid. These are the foods and drinks that we can increase in an attempt to speed things up when we are constipated. They are also, in the case of someone experiencing incomplete rectal evacuation due to soft stool consistency, the foods that we might reduce in our pursuit of a more solid and slow-moving stool.

At the top of the list of foods that make our bowel actions softer are fruits and vegetables. These days we are all well aware of the fact that too little fruit and vegetable content in our diet can make our stool consistency too hard. But it is equally true that too much fruit and vegetable content can contribute to problems associated with stools that are too soft.

Among fruits, it is grapes and stone fruit – plums, apricots and peaches – that are the most active. This applies equally to these fruits when eaten in dried form (sultanas, prunes, dried apricots and dried peaches). As a result, muesli and other fruit-containing breakfast cereals are often especially prone to make our bowels soft. Conversely, banana is the fruit that is least stimulating to the bowel. I often recommend that people add sliced banana to their breakfast cereal if they want some fruit but want to avoid the stimulating effects of too much stone fruit.

Among vegetables, there are many highly bowel-stimulating and often also flatus-inducing options. Capsicum, cabbage, onions, beans, peas, corn, brussels sprouts, lentils and chickpeas are at the top of the list. On the other hand, potato and pumpkin are the least likely vegetables to soften stool consistency or create wind.

Of course, all dietary fibre acts to draw water into our stools and thus tends to have a laxative effect. But there is a significant difference between fibre that is insoluble (nuts, fruit peel and pulp, many vegetables – in effect, things that remain 'crunchy' even when placed in liquid such as water or milk) and fibre that is soluble (bran, porridge, psyllium husks – things that are soft and that soften further when soaked in liquid). Insoluble fibre tends to be more stimulating and to encourage a more liquid 'tail' to our stools. Soluble fibre, on the other hand, tends to encourage a more bulky and formed stool.

When manipulating our dietary fibre intake to help create more solid and formed stools, a reduction in insoluble fibre intake is especially advisable. This might effectively be combined with an increase in soluble fibre intake to avoid constipation, especially in women. A good example of this sort of dietary change is to replace a breakfast of muesli with one of porridge or a breakfast cereal biscuit like Weet-Bix; to replace a salad of coleslaw with one comprising lettuce, cucumber and tomato; and to replace a summertime snack of a bunch of grapes with watermelon. This approach – replacing insoluble fibre with soluble fibre – is likely to have only a modest effect on stool consistency but is a safe first option, especially in those prone to (or especially anxious about) constipation. (Such anxiety is, understandably, much more common in women than in men, given their tendency to slower colonic transit.)

Apart from those sources of fibre contained in food, it is also appropriate to note that many people add fibre to their diets, whether in the form of soluble fibre supplements as separate entities, as additives sprinkled over food or as extra fibre added to other foods at the time of manufacture, most especially bread. For people experiencing unduly soft stool consistency, a sensible first step might be to eliminate these well-intended but unnecessary and possibly adverse supplements.

Extra fibre, however much we might have been told otherwise, really is not always an appropriate recommendation. It is not the cure of all evil, and it can be responsible for a number of unwanted side effects such as abdominal bloating and excessive flatus as well as excessively soft stools and difficulty completing rectal evacuation.

Another dietary cause of soft stools is spicy foods. Chilli, curry and garlic are at the top of this list. Spicy vegetarian food is especially likely to play havoc with stool consistency, due to the combined effect of insoluble vegetable fibre and spice.

Caffeine is another well-recognised gut stimulant. It is present in coffee, tea, cola and many energy supplements popular for their stimulant effects. Many people find that their bowels are sensitive to strong caffeinated drinks; others find that their bowel's predictable response to a strong coffee in the morning is both desirable and reassuring.

Alcoholic drinks are also apt to cause the bowel to be faster and looser. This is especially true of beer and red wine, but less so of spirits. Again, a glass or two of beer will often send us to the bathroom not only to empty our bladders but also in response to a forceful urge to empty our bowels.

Finally, the artificial sweeteners contained in so-called 'sugar-free' food and drink products are often prone to provoke both soft stools and gas. This is of particular significance to people with diabetes, people on weight-reducing diets and those who inadvertently consume these agents in sugar-free chewing gum or lollies. Many a parent has observed this effect on their child's bowel upon their return from a friend's birthday party having 'overdosed' on confectionaries of various sorts.

There are, then, many dietary causes of soft stools, and it is always worth trying to identify those things that can readily and safely be withdrawn from our diets in the pursuit of a more solid stool. Yet fruits and vegetables are vitally healthy components of virtually everyone's diet, and in many instances a reduction of these foods would be impractical (vegetarians and diabetics, in particular, rely heavily if not entirely on fruit and vegetables for their nutrition), not to mention dishearteningly unpalatable. And I know that if I, for one, were told that the only option for me to correct my excessively soft stool consistency was to reduce my intake of caffeine, spices and alcohol (especially beer), I would find that advice frankly depressing.

The good news is that there really is no need to dramatically alter your diet in order to achieve that ideal stool consistency. The medical solution is simple, safe and effective, altogether more predictable and much healthier for you than extreme dietary manipulation.

Achieving solid stool consistency through medication

Loperamide hydrochloride (also known simply as loperamide) really is the most ingenious medication. It is taken by mouth, usually in capsule or tablet form, and has an anti-diarrhoeal effect. It works by slowing down intestinal peristalsis and reducing secretions from the lining cells of our intestines. It works on the intestines in precisely the same way as do the opiate analgesic drugs codeine, morphine, oxycodone, pethidine and others.

But loperamide has two remarkable characteristics that differentiate it sharply from the opiate analgesics. First, it is barely absorbed into the bloodstream; only at extraordinarily high dosages is it absorbed in measurable amounts. Consequently, at recommended normal dosages, it causes no side effects outside the intestinal tract. So it helpfully slows down intestinal peristalsis but rarely has any systemic side effects and virtually never interferes with the absorption of any other medications you might be taking.

(Since it generally has much more effect on the large than on the small intestine, an overdose of loperamide will cause constipation first and foremost. But it can, at very high dosages, have other more serious adverse effects, so its use at high dosages must always be under medical supervision.)

The second remarkable characteristic of loperamide is that the intestines do not become adjusted to or dependent on its action. There is therefore no need for steadily rising doses over time, and there is no 'rebound' diarrhoea if it is suddenly stopped. Once you find the dose that works for you, you can confidently expect that dose to remain effective into the future. And if you do decide to stop it (or if you forget to take it with you on holidays), your bowel will return promptly to its pre-loperamide state – no better, but definitely no worse.

There is, however, one property of loperamide that requires a little care and consideration, and that is the fact that the effective dose varies greatly between individuals. Some people – especially women – with unambiguously soft stools are exquisitely sensitive to its actions, and will become constipated even at very low doses. Others, especially those who have had extensive colonic resections, will respond only to quite high doses.

The reason that this is a problem is that we doctors are used to prescribing medications within a tight dose range. It is common for any given medication to be formulated in tablets or capsules such that the standard daily dose is just one such tablet or capsule daily. And it is common for this dose to be doubled, at most, if the standard dose is ineffective. In the case of loperamide, however, the standard tablet or capsule contains two milligrams (2mg), but in many patients with unduly soft stools (more often women), just a solitary 2mg capsule per day can cause discouraging degrees of constipation. In others (more often men), a much higher daily dose of even 12mg (six 2mg capsules taken throughout the day) might prove quite ineffective.

This wide degree of variation in effective dosage means that unless you are prepared to find – under medical supervision – the dose that suits your own specific needs, you are unlikely to obtain the best result from loperamide, notwithstanding its wonderful safety even when used for a very long period of time. So let's look at how to do that.

How to get started with loperamide

In those for whom a low dose of loperamide is likely to be effective (as I have already said, this is more often the case with women, who on average have slower colonic transit times than men), I start by prescribing a specially formulated very-low-dose capsule of just

0.33mg, or one-sixth of the standard 2mg capsule. In this situation, I recommend taking just one of these 0.33mg capsules every morning for one week. After that, the patient must decide whether that very low dose is sufficient for them. If not, they should increase it to two capsules (0.66mg) taken every morning.

By very gradually increasing the dose in this manner, patients rarely become badly constipated. If they reach a daily dose of six 0.33mg capsules, they can be transferred to standard 'off the shelf' 2mg capsules, and can continue to increase their daily dose from there. The advantage of this approach is that rarely is a single 0.33 mg capsule per day sufficient to cause constipation (although I do have a small number of patients who find that even this very small dose once or twice every week achieves the desired result).

On the other hand, for people for whom I suspect that one standard 2mg capsule is probably not going to be sufficient (this is the case for most men and certainly for those people who have previously undergone extensive colonic resection), a starting dose of 2mg can be increased every week (or even a little faster) until the optimal dose is reached – that is, until the desired stool consistency has been achieved.

When using loperamide, there is no need to reduce dietary fibre intake. In fact, there can be real benefits to combining the two – the correct dose of loperamide to slow down peristalsis, and enough fibre to maintain stool bulk and form.

I simply cannot overemphasise the simplicity and safety of using loperamide to help achieve appropriately solid stool consistency. In fact, overcoming individual patients' objections that they 'don't have diarrhoea' or 'prefer to take something natural' represents the most difficult part of prescribing loperamide to improve stool consistency. Given that its use allows the person to continue eating their usual intake of fruit and vegetables, that it has no systemic side effects at standard doses and no addictive action whatsoever, and that starting and gradually increasing from a very low dose is unlikely to result in troublesome constipation, loperamide really is the smart and safe way for people suffering from excessively soft stool to achieve ideal stool consistency.

But what of people suffering from the opposite – stool that is difficult to pass? This is what we discuss in the next chapter.

5

The use of laxatives

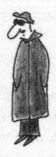

For those lucky folk who happen to be doubly blessed with speedy colonic transit and inherently effective toileting behaviours, obeying that first vital Golden Rule –to await an irresistible urge – comes all too easily. But for those of us who suffer from sluggish bowels, or whose bowel habits are beset by bad timing and counterproductive straining, that all-important, forceful urge is well beyond reach without some external assistance. And that external assistance will take the form of laxatives.

Sadly, laxatives have come to be seen as unhealthy, inevitably habit-forming and even perhaps somehow subversive. Many people who take laxatives on a regular basis are reluctant to admit this even to their doctors, let alone to their family or friends. We have created an atmosphere whereby taking laxatives on a regular basis has become something of which to be ashamed. Imagine if that applied to the taking of medications prescribed for the control of high blood pressure, diabetes or asthma! Since laxatives are the central element of the treatment of the equally valid complaint of constipation, it is ludicrous that we have allowed this situation to develop.

In these 'high-fibre times', we have been well and truly brainwashed into believing that the solution to our constipation rests entirely with dietary manipulation. By implication, we have been made to believe that the very cause of our constipation is our inadequate diet – not eating enough fruit and vegetables and fibre, and not drinking enough fluid. This really is simplistic and unhelpful. Blaming the patient for a problem not of their own making doesn't help to fix the problem, and only adds insult and self-recrimination to the frustration and physical discomfort of their condition.

Slow-colonic-transit constipation is the source of an inordinately large amount of discomfort and distress across the planet. Approximately half of the adult female population experiences regular, if not constant, problems as a result of it: difficulty with rectal evacuation, infrequent rectal evacuation, straining to evacuate, abdominal bloating, discomfort, anxiety and even misery. And slow-colonic-transit constipation is a chronic – that is, ongoing – condition, just like high blood pressure or diabetes or asthma. Like these conditions, it can rarely if ever be cured outright. And so, just like other chronic complaints, it needs to be managed in an ongoing manner.

What people with slow-colonic-transit constipation need from their health carers is a strategy to assist them to manage their lifelong condition. They need assistance that will enable them to reach the bathroom with an irresistible urge. What they do not need is to be told that the cause of their problems is their own inadequate diet or lack of fluid intake or even lack of physical exercise. And the simple and reliable way to enable them to obey that first and most important Golden Rule is with the aid of laxatives.

Types of laxatives

Let's accept, then, that laxatives are neither poisonous nor pre-cancerous, neither illegal nor immoral. And let's also accept that, for people with ongoing constipation, the reality is simple – laxatives are essential for the control of the unpleasant symptoms caused by their constipation.

But there are many different types of laxatives, and some are not ideal for long-term use. This is usually because these laxatives tend to result in the bowel becoming dependent on them, with the need, over time, for steadily increasing doses of the same laxative to provoke the same response. Other laxatives are undesirable because they provoke a lot of gas production, which can be both uncomfortable and embarrassing, while still others are unpleasant to taste or just plain difficult to swallow.

There are four main subgroups of laxatives, each of which we'll look at now.

Fibre supplements and water-binding gums

Soluble fibre supplements are almost always the first laxatives people try. They are not habit-forming, and they are generally only mildly active. They include natural bran, psyllium husks, wheat pectin, flax seed and others.

These laxatives work by absorbing water into the fibre, which swells and remains within the bulk of the stool. The result is a bulkier stool with a more banana-like shape, which stretches the intestine from within, provoking contractions and stimulating faster colonic transit. They also encourage the production of gas once the fibre-filled stool reaches the large intestine and is exposed to the action of the local bacterial population. As a result, they tend to provoke uncomfortable abdominal bloating and an awkward excess of flatus.

Fibre supplements can also be difficult for some people to ingest. They have a naturally grainy and gritty texture, which makes them difficult to swallow. They can be dissolved in water to form a gel-like consistency, sprinkled over food (usually breakfast cereal) or mixed into a 'smoothie' for ease of swallowing. As they are flavourless, the absence of taste and the awkward consistency have encouraged the production of commercial preparations that include artificial flavouring (orange seems to be the most popular). Some commercial preparations come in capsule form, but since a standard dose of soluble fibre (usually about 5g) corresponds to about eight or nine capsules, this option tends to be inordinately expensive.

In practice, fibre supplements are weak laxatives that tend to have a much more pronounced effect on the bowel function of people with normal colonic transit. Men – who generally have normal or fast colonic transit – often note significant changes in bowel form and function when they start taking fibre supplements. Women with true slow-colonic-transit constipation, however, are likely to experience disproportionate bloating with little real improvement in their constipation.

In short, fibre supplements are much more popular among prescribers (doctors and pharmacists, who like their non-habit-forming and generally benign health benefits) than among constipated women (who dislike the bloating and are desperate for something that actually works).

Water-binding gums include guar gum and xanthan gum. These also bind water, although they do so even more intensely than most fibre supplements. As a result, they tend to swell more dramatically when exposed to water. They have the same issue of difficulty with ingestion, and they cannot be safely encapsulated for fear of their becoming transiently lodged in the lower oesophagus, where they might conceivably expand rapidly and stretch or even rupture the oesophagus.

There is little current interest in the use of water-binding gums in the treatment of constipation. Nevertheless, they have many of the same properties of the soluble fibre supplements but with a lesser tendency to provoke flatus. Thus they might rise again in the treatment of constipation at some stage.

Lubricant oils

Many oils have a laxative action. Liquid paraffin is perhaps the best known and most widely available of these. It is essentially tasteless, although it is often prepared commercially with chocolate or other flavourings.

Oils have little effect on the consistency or composition of the stool itself, but instead tend to coat the intestinal lining and act as lubricants, easing the passage of the stool through the intestine. They are, therefore, mild laxatives with little impact in people with established slow colonic transit. They are often effective in the management of milder degrees of constipation, especially in children. They are not habit-forming, but they tend to leave an oily residue after a bowel action, and some people describe an annoying oily leakage after defecation.

It is important to distinguish between paraffin oil and the well-known but old-fashioned (and now rarely used) castor oil. The latter, although an oil, is also a direct intestinal stimulant, which makes it not only a much more powerful laxative than paraffin oil but a habit-forming one as well. Hence, it is much less suitable for ongoing use. What's more, it has a particularly unpleasant taste.

Herbal and manufactured stimulant laxatives

Many naturally occurring herbs – including senna and cascara – have a laxative action. These are powerful and, at least initially, predictably effective laxatives. They work by chemically stimulating the intestine's muscle tube to contract. As a result, they provoke intestinal contractions whether or not the intestine contains any faecal matter. From an intestinal point of view, this is not at all 'natural', since it is the distension of the intestinal wall by the contents of the intestine that results in natural bowel contractions.

Manufactured stimulant laxatives – bisacodyl is easily the most widely used – have similar properties and are equally popular. Like herbal laxatives they are often presented in tablet form, making them exceptionally palatable. But also like herbal laxatives, their mechanism of action is to directly provoke intestinal contractions, which can translate into painful intestinal cramps.

Even worse, both herbal and manufactured stimulant laxatives have the unfortunate tendency to induce tachyphylaxis. This is the technical term for physiological tolerance, or the steadily reducing response to these agents with repeated use over time. Longstanding users of these laxatives, especially those who have used them once or twice every day for prolonged periods, often report the need for steadily rising doses to maintain the usual response. I have looked after patients who had resorted to taking upwards of 50 tablets in search of a response.

I think it is fair to describe these agents as potentially addictive. Although stopping them suddenly does not result in any obvious 'withdrawal' reaction, people in this situation are unlikely to be able to have a spontaneous bowel action, and will almost always need to take some other laxative (if not the herbal/manufactured stimulant agent itself) to get their bowels working again.

Just the same, on a worldwide scale, these are far and away the most commonly prescribed laxatives. Their popularity is built largely on their small tablet presentation and the initially predictable response to each dose.

Herbal laxatives are especially popular, because of their claim to be 'natural'. While it is true that senna, cascara and the other herbal laxatives are indeed naturally occurring, this is also true of little red berries and oleander leaves. Just because something grows naturally on the roadside or can be plucked from a thriving plant in an untouched rainforest does not make it safe (let alone advisable) to eat. The herbal pharmaceuticals industry gains great traction from the 'natural' branding of its products, which in the case of herbal laxatives is at best misleading, and perhaps even mischievous.

This is not to say that herbal and manufactured stimulant laxatives are poisonous or carcinogenic, or that it isn't often possible to wean people off these agents and replace them with laxatives that are more appropriate for long-term use. But I cannot support the instigation of 'new' laxative therapy using any agent that I know will inherently make its user more and more reliant on it and less and less likely to achieve spontaneous bowel contractions.

Sure, if a person is already dependent on these laxatives but is managing satisfactorily, it is fair and reasonable to let them continue. This is especially appropriate in elderly people, who might argue that they haven't got long enough to go in life to warrant the disruption associated with a change to their laxative regime. But in the vast majority of cases, it is sensible to encourage people to move away from herbal and stimulant laxatives in search of a return to at least some spontaneous bowel activity, and far better still not to have started them on potentially 'addictive' laxatives in the first place.

Osmotic laxatives

This family of laxatives includes both salts and sugars of a type that are not readily absorbed by the intestine. In other words, when these salts or sugars are swallowed, they are not absorbed through the intestinal wall and into the bloodstream but remain inside the stomach, small intestine and large intestine.

Perhaps the best known of these is Epsom salts. Whereas common table salt (sodium chloride) is quickly absorbed into the bloodstream, the intestines are incapable of absorbing Epsom salts (magnesium sulfate). Both the magnesium and the sulfate components remain inside the stomach and intestines. Similarly, whereas standard white table sugar, which is made more or less of pure glucose, is absorbed promptly into the bloodstream, the intestines are incapable of absorbing the commonly used artificial sweetener sorbitol, so it too remains inside the stomach and intestines.

The effect of these salts or sugars remaining inside the intestines is that they rapidly achieve an excessive concentration within the intestine, which the body recognises and immediately seeks to correct. Since it cannot draw these sorts of salts or sugars out from the intestine and into the bloodstream in order to equalise their concentration within the intestine with that of the bloodstream, the body must instead transfer water from the bloodstream back into the intestine to dilute that salt or sugar, equalising the concentration that way. The practical result of swallowing Epsom salts or sorbitol, therefore, is the rapid inflow of water from the bloodstream into the stomach and small intestine.

This entry of water into the upper intestine creates a large column of liquid that stretches the intestinal wall and provokes the bowel wall to contract – much like the effect of a soluble fibre supplement, only much more rapid and substantial. Under the influence of the peristaltic contraction waves it has provoked, this column of liquid passes rapidly through the intestines, water being added all the way until the concentration is equalised. The end result is a watery bowel action arriving at speed; evacuation can be urgent and should produce complete emptying of the large intestine.

Osmotic laxatives are not habit-forming, since they induce intestinal contractions in a physiological manner. However, the salts are often unpalatable, and even the sugars can be quite sickly and difficult to ingest. Further, the sugars (but not the salts) are associated with prominent gas production due to the action of colonic bacteria, which is quite a disincentive for their use.

For an effective result, large doses of osmotic agents are generally required, especially in people with significant slow-colonic-transit constipation. Nevertheless, their cleansing action and the absence of any habit-forming tendency make osmotic laxatives the laxatives of choice for all but the most minor degrees of constipation. More on osmotic laxatives shortly.

Powerful laxatives and the 'all or nothing' effect

A person suffering from longstanding constipation might well dream of nothing more than having a spontaneous, effortless and truly satisfying bowel action, resulting in a magnificent, perfectly formed stool. In the imagination of such a person, the ideal output of their laxative dose might be precisely such a textbook stool – something they could almost plate up and proudly show off to friends and family.

But the reality is quite different. In response to taking a powerful laxative of the herbal, manufactured stimulant or osmotic varieties, people with sluggish bowels tend to exhibit an 'all or nothing' response. By this I mean that, with a small dose, there is little response. With a slightly larger dose, still nothing seems to happen. But when the effective dose is finally reached, the bowel's response tends to be voluminous and vigorous, urgent and even overwhelming – not at all that textbook result for which they had been hoping.

For anyone with constipation of even a moderate degree – certainly, for anyone with constipation of a severity sufficient to warrant the use of these strong laxatives – the prospect of producing a textbook stool in response to the use of any of these laxatives is a distant one indeed. The almost inevitable result of an effective dose of a herbal, manufactured stimulant or osmotic laxative is a forceful, urgent, semi-formed, even liquid stool.

This is an important point to appreciate, because the generally recommended pursuit of the ideal, beautifully formed stool can mislead people suffering from constipation into believing that this result is both achievable and necessary in their case, when in fact it is rarely either. The incorrect belief that the proper outcome of the correct dose of laxatives must be a fully formed stool only discourages sufferers from using these strong laxatives at the dose they really do need.

This is not to say that people with constipation who require strong laxatives can never achieve a well-formed stool. It's just that they cannot do so in response to taking strong laxatives – strong laxatives taken at effective doses cause urgent, loose stools, even in those with sluggish bowels. That's just the way it is. Strong laxatives can, however, be used to restore spontaneous bowel activity and to help achieve spontaneous and well-formed bowel actions. It all depends on which laxatives you use and how you use them.

The case for laxative use

I hope that you can now appreciate the following points in favour of judicious and medically supervised laxative use:

- For people with slow-colonic-transit constipation, laxatives are the essential element of treatment. Dietary intervention alone is rarely sufficient, and increasing dietary fibre intake often aggravates abdominal bloating. Discouraging constipated people from taking laxatives is unhelpful and, frankly, cruel.
- Osmotic laxatives of the salt variety are the best laxatives from the perspective of not being habit-

forming as well as having less tendency to produce excessive gas. Osmotic laxatives of the sugar variety are also safe and not habit-forming, but are associated with excessive gas production. Herbal and manufactured stimulant laxatives are strong and easy to take, but are habit-forming and become progressively less effective the longer they are used.

- Powerful laxatives – whether herbal, manufactured stimulant or osmotic – are required for the effective treatment of all but the mildest degrees of constipation. However, they generally do not work at low doses, and an effective dose commonly results in an all-or-nothing response – a powerful cleansing of the bowel rather than the production of a well-formed stool. It is therefore important to use them correctly – as outlined later in this chapter.

So which are the best laxatives?

This is a really sensitive question. Individual sufferers and individual prescribers will have their own favourites. In providing you with mine, I ask you to consider your own circumstances – which laxatives you have been using already, and for how long – and to consult with your own trusted doctor or pharmacist before making any changes.

In my practice, I regularly recommend the following agents:

- *Magnesium salts*   These include the time-honoured Epsom salts (magnesium sulfate) and magnesium oxide, as well as many others which I do not generally prescribe. They come as powders or even crystals, which should be dissolved in water and disguised in juice or cordial because of their intensely bitter taste. Chilling the solution will also reduce the intensity of the unpleasant flavour. Encapsulation of magnesium sulfate has been tried, which results in a highly effective laxative and is especially advantageous as a means of eliminating the bad taste, as well as a means of providing a more accurate and reproducible dosage.

- *Macrogol 3350*   This also belongs to the osmotic family, but is more palatable than magnesium salts. It is also a little less potent; however, once the effective dose has been reached, macrogol works every bit as well as magnesium salts. It is a very popular agent, but is often prescribed at inadequately low dosage and unnecessarily high frequency. A weekly cleanse is the most that should be required.

- *Magnesium oxide + sodium picosulfate*   Known as the 'nuclear laxative', this is a combination of an osmotic laxative (magnesium oxide) and a stimulant agent (sodium picosulfate), and is often prescribed to achieve bowel preparation before a colonoscopy. It offers reliably intense bowel cleansing, but is regarded as unpalatable by many people. The stimulant component is also potentially habit-forming – although, to be fair, when taken no more often than once per week this is an exceptionally unlikely prospect. This is the most powerful agent in my laxative armoury, and its reliability at the standard dose (two sachets, taken three to four hours apart) makes it a trusted weapon.

How to use laxatives

Here's where that difference between the sexes comes into play.

As we've already discussed, there is a significant difference, on average, between the bowel functions of men and women – with men tending to be 'fast and fruity' and women to be 'slow and sluggish'. However, not appreciating these physiological differences, many men develop a misguided sense of their own superiority and assume that women suffering from constipation are doing something wrong. I have spoken to scores of constipated women in the presence of their husbands or male partners, and have observed firsthand the deeply but quite incorrectly held belief among many of these men that there is a straightforward solution to be had by their partners in the form of some relatively simple diet or lifestyle change. Alas, since many prescribers – doctors and pharmacists alike – are also men, they too can be invested in this erroneous and ultimately unhelpful attitude. Since the average male's experience involves spontaneous and at least daily bowel actions – often in the morning – we male prescribers have come to prescribe laxatives only under sufferance, and often as a last resort. And, when we do, we routinely prescribe them on a once- or twice-daily basis.

We seem irreversibly committed to this notion of daily laxative use. However, since:

- almost all sufferers of ongoing constipation require strong laxatives to have a meaningful response,
- effective doses of these strong laxatives cause frequent, liquid bowel actions, and
- it is far too draining and time-consuming to clean the bowel out like this day after day,

the result is that we tend to prescribe these laxatives at ineffectively low doses, yet still on a daily basis.

Consequently, people using laxatives in this manner either do not achieve the all-important complete bowel emptying that would be associated with true relief from their symptoms or do not achieve the anticipated daily bowel action. This accounts for the widespread dissatisfaction with laxative treatment schedules reported by a very large percentage of longstanding laxative users.

In fact, if we are to move towards a more effective laxative regime, we really need to abandon this male-centred narrative. What we need to do is to accept that the frequency with which we open our bowels is simply not as important – in fact, it is nowhere near as important – as how easily and completely we empty our bowels when we do have a bowel action.

As observed at the beginning of this book, when all is said and done, it is the ease and completeness, and not the frequency, of bowel emptying that really matters. A totally empty bowel is the desired outcome of any bowel action, the Holy Grail of bowel function, the very reason for obeying those three Golden Rules. The end result of every satisfying bowel action is an empty bowel, and the basis of every satisfactory bowel habit is the ability to regularly and reliably empty the bowel completely. And for people with constipation, this is most appropriately achieved by using a cleansing dose of an osmotic laxative of the salt variety.

But since these sorts of bowel clean-outs are often time-consuming and even draining, they cannot – and need not – be repeated daily. They are generally best taken just once a week, or even less frequently. Many people with genuinely slow colonic transit will experience days, even a week or more of sustained comfort after thoroughly emptying their bowels in this manner. And many will experience the return of spontaneous bowel actions – often after years of apparent laxative dependence – after achieving only a few such clean-outs just one week apart.

Over time, spontaneous and effective bowel activity can be maintained, possibly for many weeks, after a single cleansing dose of an osmotic laxative, allowing the gap between doses to be gradually extended. A strict initial strategy of once-weekly laxative use can often be superseded by just an occasional clean-out, allowing not only for relief from bloating, straining and discomfort but also for much more flexibility in lifestyle and a greater individual sense of control over their own bodies.

How to get started – and how to keep going

In my experience, it takes about four or five weeks for most people to arrive at the best dose and the best timing of that dose for their own purposes. Since getting the bowels totally cleaned out is the aim of this strategy, it is better to take too much laxative and be 'too clean' than it is to take too little and not be clean enough. As a result, it is often the case that people starting this regime will tend to overdose in the first few weeks as they gradually identify their 'ideal' dose.

Similar to the situation described in Chapter 4 with respect to the anti-diarrhoeal medication loperamide, there is a wide range of effective laxative dosages among people suffering with constipation. Each person will respond differently, and it is not always possible to anticipate who will respond briskly or slowly and who will require small or large doses to do so.

It is important to start by understanding the following:

- You cannot be sure when you begin this process how much you will need to take to achieve a thoroughly emptied bowel.
- You will nevertheless need to take enough to ensure that you have cleaned out your bowel.
- You will need to adjust the dose on a weekly basis until you find your own predictably effective dose.
- You will need to persevere, since immediate improvement, although possible, is not usual, and many weeks, occasionally months, are required to appreciate the full benefit.

I generally recommend the following sequence:

1. Select the day of the week that will best be dedicated to the process of cleaning out your bowel. This is often a weekend day, for obvious reasons. For the sake of this example, let's use Saturday.
2. On Friday night, take one standard dose (let's use macrogol as an example, for which one standard dose is two sachets) at about 10 pm.
3. What you do next will depend on your response to that first dose.
   a. If you experience an emphatic cleansing response to this dose overnight or first thing the next morning, this is unequivocally good news (although an uncommon occurrence, in my

experience). Sure, you will have had a disturbed night's sleep, but you now know that you respond briskly and effectively to a low dose, which you can continue to take in the same manner next Friday night. Alternatively, you can delay taking the next week's dose until the Saturday morning, avoiding the overnight disturbance but confident that you will have responded to it by Saturday night.

b. If you experience no such response – only a minor response or none at all – you should repeat the standard dose (two sachets) at 8 am on Saturday.

c. If you still don't respond (or respond only minimally), you should repeat the standard dose at 10 am on Saturday, and again every two hours until a response commences. Although it is always better to be 'too clean' than not clean enough, once your bowel starts to work you should not continue to take any more laxatives – even if the first bowel action is solid. If you do, you are likely to take too much laxative and end up sore and spent. It is always likely that the first week's response will be more prolonged and more complete (as well as more draining), so there is no need to overdo it by taking more laxatives once your bowel has started to work.

4. Each week, you should adjust the dose and the timing of that dose until you find the best balance for yourself. Some people find that splitting the dose between Friday night and Saturday morning (or

whichever days you choose) works best for them; others prefer to take the entire dose in the morning. Some find that they respond to a single standard dose, while others require five or more for effect. You will simply have to try to see for yourself.

5. You must persevere to get the most out of this strategy. After months, years or even decades of constipation, an immediate correction cannot be expected; time is required to see whether this strategy is going to be effective for you. The initial response or two can be uncomfortable and even painful, especially if your constipation is generally associated with painful abdominal cramps or bloating. If you expect an instant miracle and are not prepared to persevere, you will never find out whether this strategy would have been effective for you.

6. In general, six to ten weekly doses are required to confidently establish your individual pattern. Usually, by this time, spontaneous bowel actions have recommenced between doses. If you are experiencing daily spontaneous and effective bowel actions, it is understandably difficult to convince yourself to take a cleansing dose of laxatives 'just because it's Saturday'. In fact, once your bowel is working this well, you can comfortably reduce the frequency of your doses to once every two weeks. I prefer this to stopping the strategy altogether. In time, however, as the days or even weeks pass since your last laxative dose, you will be able to recognise the slowing down

of colonic transit and the return of the symptoms of constipation for which another cleansing dose is appropriate. This regime of occasional bowel cleansing is the most common long-term pattern of laxative use among my patients.

As much as constipated people might wish to experience a totally spontaneous, fully autonomous bowel habit characterised by completely effortless, entirely satisfying and perfectly formed bowel actions – in short, a permanent cure – this is only rarely possible. Even with the optimal use of non-habit-forming laxatives as outlined above, that inherent propensity to slow colonic transit is never likely to disappear completely.

In other words, even if spontaneous bowel actions have been restored by the use of weekly (and then occasional) cleansing with osmotic laxatives, once you stop taking these laxatives altogether, the symptoms of constipation are likely to return over time. Slow-colonic-transit constipation is, after all, a chronic complaint no different in that respect from other chronic complaints such as high blood pressure or diabetes. A total and permanent cure is an unreasonable expectation, meaning that ongoing management will always be required.

6

Other medications that affect the bowel

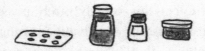

Many medications commonly prescribed for a wide range of afflictions can affect our bowels. While it would be impossible to list here every medication that does so – especially since different people are affected differently by the same medications – there are a few that appear consistently to cause either loose and frequent stools or the reverse.

The following lists are necessarily incomplete, but will be of interest to many people since these medications are in such common use. Before you read these lists, however, it is important for you to appreciate two points:

- If you already have a tendency towards loose stools, medications that tend to cause loose stools are more likely to aggravate the problem. Likewise, if you are already prone to constipation, you can expect that medications with that side effect will make your constipation worse.
- Just because a particular medication might cause disturbances in bowel function, this is no reason to avoid or stop using that medication. The medication will have been prescribed for good reason, and any consequent disturbance of bowel function can nearly always be well managed by the judicious use of loperamide (if you are loose) or osmotic laxatives (if you are constipated). This will allow you to benefit from the original medication without continuing to experience the undesired bowel consequences. In general, your medications are more important to your health than are any bowel disturbances they might cause.

Medications that cause loose, frequent stools

- *Metformin and other oral hypoglycaemic medications* These drugs are used to lower blood sugar levels in the treatment of diabetes, and commonly provoke loose stools and diarrhoea.
- *Non-steroidal anti-inflammatory drugs (NSAIDs)* This is a huge family of painkilling medications used for joint and muscle pain, menstrual pain, headache and almost every other sort of pain. Ibuprofen, naproxen, indomethacin and diclofenac are among

the most common, but there are a dozen or more different NSAIDs in common use.

- *Antibiotics* While antibiotics are used to treat infection in all parts of the body, their use can also result in the eradication of normal intestinal bacteria. A common consequence of this can be diarrhoea, which settles promptly once the course of antibiotics has been completed or discontinued. In less common circumstances, this suppression of the usual bacterial population paves the way for the overgrowth of otherwise inconsequential bacteria which, when they multiply in large numbers, can cause serious inflammation and ulceration of the large intestine. Antibiotic-associated diarrhoea is common, and occasionally serious.

- *Colchicine* This medication is used primarily in the treatment of gout (a form of arthritis), but has also been shown to be of benefit in patients with coronary heart disease. Diarrhoea is a common adverse effect that can limit its usefulness in these patients.

Medications that cause constipation

- *Painkillers of the opiate family* Codeine, morphine, pethidine, oxycodone and fentanyl all cause constipation, by directly slowing intestinal motility. In fact, this is exactly the same action as that of loperamide, as described in Chapter 4. People who have undergone painful surgery are almost always prescribed these medications; constipation is an extremely common problem after major surgery, especially for people already predisposed to slow colonic transit.

- *Tricyclic antidepressant medications* Although in less common use these days, the tricyclic antidepressant medications (amitriptyline, imipramine) remain extremely effective in the treatment of depression and chronic pain syndromes. Among other side effects, they commonly cause constipation.

- *Benztropine* Commonly used in the treatment of Parkinson's disease, this medication can aggravate the constipation that is often an inherent aspect of the condition itself.

- *Iron supplements* These are extremely widely prescribed, especially during and immediately after pregnancy. They are famous for causing constipation and are now often combined with other agents designed to counter their constipating effects.

- *Calcium supplements* Calcium supplementation for osteoporosis is an especially commonly prescribed mineral supplement, and often provokes or exacerbates constipation. Calcium is also often a component of antacid preparations (used in the treatment of indigestion and gastro-oesophageal reflux), which explains why some of these preparations also cause constipation.

- *Calcium channel-blocking drugs* Used in the treatment of high blood pressure, calcium channel-blocking drugs such as verapamil are also known to contribute to constipation. Other members of this family of drugs in more common use in the treatment of high blood pressure – amlodipine, lercanidipine and diltiazem – are a little less likely to cause constipation.

- *SSRI (and related) antidepressant medications* This very large family of medications is in extremely widespread use worldwide for the treatment of depression, anxiety and related mental health problems. These are excellent medications that have made an enormous difference to millions of people and have also helped to reduce the social stigma so often associated with mental health problems. From a gastrointestinal perspective, nausea is easily the most common adverse effect, but all of these medications can also cause either diarrhoea or constipation. Those that are a little more likely to cause diarrhoea include sertraline, fluvoxamine, fluoxetine and venlafaxine. Those that are a little more likely to cause constipation include paroxetine, fluvoxamine and mirtazapine. Overall, fluvoxamine appears to be associated with the most gastrointestinal disturbance; citalopram and escitalopram appear to be the best tolerated from this perspective.

Remember, the medications you have been prescribed are almost certainly important – possibly even absolutely essential – for your general health. So, while they may indeed interfere with the workings of your bowel, that interference does not mean that you should stop taking them. Please consult with your doctor, who will be able to advise you as to whether your bowel disturbance is due to your medication, whether there might be equally effective alternative medications that are less likely to have the same impact on your bowel or, if you simply must continue to take these medications, how you might best correct the negative consequences on your bowel these essential medications are having.

7

Alternative treatments: faecal transplants, probiotics, enemas and colonic irrigation

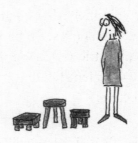

There are many reasons why bowel-related conditions attract some strange and in some cases unproven therapies. Certainly people are often embarrassed by their bowel problems, regarding them either as unworthy of bringing to the attention of – or just too awkward to discuss with – their family doctor or pharmacist. Alternatively, having summoned the courage to raise the issue with their GP or pharmacist, they might have found that their complaint was not paid appropriate attention or was not taken sufficiently seriously, or that the advice offered was simply ineffective. And since many of these complaints are longstanding and, by inference, do not represent a serious threat to the sufferer, a common attitude is: 'If it isn't going to kill me, why bother bringing it to my doctor's attention?'

So people with bowel problems might readily turn to alternative therapies and alternative therapists, with whom they might feel less awkward or by whom they might feel they will be taken more seriously. While the simple act of taking an interest and showing care builds trust and can be genuinely therapeutic, many people with bowel-related problems seem happy to embark on treatments that have little rational physiological basis, let alone any credible scientific support to indicate that they might be effective.

However, there are some specific alternative treatments that are genuinely topical and deserve a little more careful analysis.

Faecal transplants

The notion of having someone else's faeces introduced directly into your own bowel is initially both repugnant and somehow laughable. The intention of such a strange concept, however, is not to introduce faeces so much as to inoculate the recipient's bowel with the literally millions of microorganisms (mainly bacteria) contained within that faeces.

This emerging treatment reflects the growing appreciation in mainstream medical thinking of the importance to bowel health – and to our health more broadly – of the bowel's bacterial milieu. To be absolutely clear, however, the solidly established indications for so-called 'faecal microbial transplantation' are currently very limited.

There are some people whose loss of normal faecal microbial balance makes them susceptible to the overgrowth of a serious and potentially very harmful organism called *Clostridium difficile* (of which there are numerous strains and subtypes). In people who suffer repeated bouts of *Clostridium difficile* gastroenteritis, there is now good evidence to support treatment by faecal microbial transplantation, and this treatment is increasingly being offered by established mainstream medical experts.

Over time, other indications for faecal microbial transplantation are likely to emerge. Currently the impact on the body's overall immune system of the bowel's bacterial environment is being especially closely examined. In time, faecal microbial transplantation might come to be seen as an effective treatment for conditions that do not at first appear to be connected to the bowel.

For now, however, the need for caution and common sense is especially great. We do not yet know which specific bacteria are missing in those people who might benefit from faecal microbial transplantation, and we do not know which specific bacteria are the ones that need to be replaced. In truth, we have no idea whose faeces contains the bacteria that make for a good donor and whose do not.

This is definitely a case of 'watch this space'. However, while many desperate bowel-disorder sufferers continue to seek what they hope might be a magic cure through unproven treatments, I can say with confidence that people suffering right now from the sorts of bowel disorders described in this book are not likely – now or in the near future – to be suitable recipients of faecal microbial transplantation.

Our desire to be decisively cured is a powerful one. It makes us consider taking potentially harmful drugs, undergoing potentially dangerous surgery and embarking on unequivocally unproven therapies. Often, however, it is a better strategy to persevere with much more basic management techniques in appreciation of the reality that these problems can only be managed on a daily basis rather than cured once and for all.

Probiotics

Probiotics are actually microorganisms – mostly bacteria. Probiotic capsules contain millions of these bacteria that are swallowed in the hope that they will make it all the way down to our bowel, where they will either replace important bacteria that are missing, or will displace potentially harmful bacteria that are doing us no good. They are widely available and, like so many 'over the counter' bowel treatments, they are essentially harmless but largely ineffective.

Probiotics are most likely to be effective in reducing the severity of antibiotic-associated diarrhoea. Diarrhoea is a common consequence of taking antibiotics, and this is likely to be due to the unwanted imbalance in the colonic bacterial milieu that results from the action of the antibiotics on the normal colonic bacterial population. Other therapeutic claims – and probiotics have been proposed as a treatment for a wide variety of conditions – are more or less totally unproven, and are certainly not regarded as acceptable by regulatory authorities.

As in the case of faecal microbial transplantation, we simply do not yet know which specific microorganisms and which specific probiotic preparations are the 'good' ones. We do not even know for sure whether commercially available probiotic preparations are better than natural yoghurt, which is another rich source of these microorganisms.

All in all, probiotics are insufficiently proven and grossly overprescribed. The appeal of a pseudoscientific explanation and the lure of a magical cure need to be balanced against the simple truth of whether or not they are reducing your symptoms. If they are, well and good. If they are not, save yourself the cost and concentrate on strategies that might actually help you.

Enemas and colonic irrigation

As previously stated, an empty bowel is a happy bowel, and the ultimate objective of every bowel action is to get the bowel empty. For those who are unable to achieve this spontaneously, a thorough emptying can be achieved by taking a decisive dose of laxatives, preferably of the osmotic variety.

But why not empty the bowel by administration of an enema, you might ask? Actually, this represents an entirely rational approach, even if it is not quite as effective (and, often, nowhere near as acceptable) as the appropriate use of laxatives.

I regard cleaning the bowel out from below to be an important strategy to apply in certain clinical circumstances, and a useful alternative approach where standard laxative regimes are ineffective or intolerable. But let's be quite clear: the widespread notion that colonic irrigation techniques work by 'clearing out toxins' is utter nonsense. Colonic irrigation is all about the mechanical cleansing of the bowel – getting the lower bowel empty.

Commercially available enemas are generally quite low in volume when compared to rectal irrigation, which can involve 500 ml of fluid or more. They can effectively clean out the rectum and, sometimes, the lower sigmoid colon. This leaves most of the colon untouched and, all too often, persistently loaded with faeces. For people with generally normal bowel function who find themselves constipated as a result of one-off events (such as taking constipating medications, a period of immobility or a marked change of diet), an enema can be an effective one-off solution.

For others, whose predominant bowel problems relate to their inability to effect rectal emptying (but whose colonic transit is normal or very nearly normal), these enemas can be used on a more regular basis to good effect. However, they are unlikely to be more effective than self-administered rectal irrigation, which is both more flexible to administer and cheaper in the long term.

Rectal self-irrigation requires specific but very easy training from a qualified therapist, most often a nurse with appropriate expertise and experience. It involves the instillation through a simple rectal tube of a volume of warm tap water, which can vary from 200 ml to one litre depending on the underlying clinical issue and the result of some trial and error. It can be self-administered on a daily basis (most patients use it last thing at night) or less frequently depending on patient preference.

In my practice, it is used most often for those patients suffering difficulty with bowel function after surgery for rectal cancer, where the rectum has been surgically removed and part of the colon has been used to make a new junction with the lower rectum or upper anus. Unfortunately, try as it might, the colon can never recreate the specialised function of a normal, intact rectum, and these patients frequently experience urgency, frequency, difficulty completing rectal emptying and even faecal leakage and incontinence.

In this specialised group of patients, rectal self-irrigation can be life-changing. To be honest, however, it is nowhere near as popular a treatment technique among the majority of my patients, most of whom have not had surgery on their bowels. Nevertheless, rectal self-irrigation has real merit as an option, especially for those whose bowel problems relate more to the emptying of the rectum than to the slowness of their colonic transit.

So where does this leave colonic lavage – the commercially available rectal irrigation technique administered on an occasional basis in purpose-specific colonic lavage clinics by registered nurses? In general, these clinics are safe and caring environments, but they are expensive. Many patients find them very agreeable – the therapists spend time with them, they are invariably gentle and genuinely interested in their bowel complaints, and the cleansing of their bowel that follows the lavage often provides considerable symptomatic relief.

On the other hand, these visits can be time-consuming, must be fitted into the patient's weekly schedule of events, and rapidly become costly given the ongoing nature of the bowel complaint and the real need for ongoing management. Self-irrigation offers much more flexibility in terms of the 'when and where', and is vastly less expensive.

My view is that colonic lavage clinics do serve a genuinely useful purpose, and I have also recommended rectal self-irrigation more and more over the course of my career. For those people who have benefited from attending colonic lavage clinics, there is no pressing need to do otherwise. On the other hand, conversion to rectal self-irrigation is generally a sensible and straightforward alternative.

8

The relationship between bowel and brain

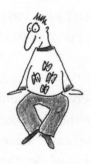

That there is a close link between the workings of our brain and those of our bowel is both common knowledge and common experience. Who hasn't experienced 'butterflies in their stomach' when anxious or excited, or the abdominal cramps and loose, urgent stools that can precede stressful situations such as public speaking or a sporting competition?

Of course, everyone responds differently to stress. For some it manifests as headache; for others as abdominal or gastrointestinal symptoms; for others still as agitation or sleep disturbance. But some sort of bowel disturbance is an unequivocally common consequence of emotional stress.

Ironically, gastrointestinal disturbance is often also a significant *cause* of stress. This can result in a powerful vicious circle in which stress – let's say, at the prospect of a job interview – provokes urgency and loose stools. In turn, the worrying prospect of experiencing another urgent bowel action that could interfere with the start of the interview can cause sufficient stress to provoke precisely such an urgent bowel action at precisely the worst possible time.

The connection between emotional stress and bowel dysfunction is complex. In general, those prone to active bowels will experience even more urgency when under stress, while those prone to sluggish bowels are likely to note exacerbation of their constipation.

But it is not always that simple. I recall a patient of mine – I'll call her Sue – with longstanding, severe and objectively proven slow-colonic-transit constipation. She was in her mid-40s, and testing of her bowel function – during which the passage of a radioactive 'meal' around her bowel had been monitored daily – had revealed that none of the ingested meal had been expelled after eight days. Sue's bowels were exceptionally sluggish, and she had been more or less totally dependent on laxatives to effect any bowel action whatsoever for 20 years or more.

Remarkably, however, Sue described how, should her father call her by telephone from his home in a distant Australian city, she would never be able to complete the phone call because of the sudden arrival of an overwhelmingly urgent need to open her bowel.

Sue's relationship with her father was strained and complex, and these very occasional and generally unexpected phone calls clearly provoked strong emotions and a correspondingly strong gastrointestinal response. Her case acts as a reminder of the very real but occasionally unpredictable association that exists between emotions, stress and bowel function.

This connection needn't always be quite so dramatic. Another patient of mine – I'll call him Brian – experienced a typically active male bowel habit for the first 50 years of his life, characterised by a predictably strong urge and an effective bowel action more or less every morning. His elevation to manager of his department at work at the age of 50 was well deserved, and he undoubtedly had the necessarily skills to assume this leadership position. He was also unequivocally highly regarded by both his team and his superiors. But the new role came with a significant increase in responsibility, and a dramatic rise in his personal stress levels.

In Brian's case, this manifested in what was, at first, a subtle change in his toileting behaviour. His working day as manager started earlier than previously, and he became a little fixated on ensuring that he had opened his bowel before he left home each day. As a result, he began to sit on the toilet every morning, before his usually strong and natural urge to open his bowel had arrived.

Since the urge to go when he reached the bathroom was now sub-optimal (a classic case of premature defecation), and since he did not want to risk being late for work, Brian would voluntarily strain to initiate rectal emptying. This was uncomfortable and often ineffective; rectal evacuation was generally incomplete, leaving him feeling dissatisfied and frustrated.

Over time, Brian opted to visit the bathroom earlier and earlier in the hope that giving the exercise more time would allow him to achieve more complete rectal emptying. In reality, however, all that happened was that he got to the bathroom more and more prematurely, with an ever-less-adequate urge to evacuate. He spent more and more time achieving less and less complete rectal emptying. Sitting and straining for lengthy periods of time resulted in the development of haemorrhoids, causing bleeding and protrusion – which was the reason Brian's doctor referred him to see me.

But Brian's main complaint was that he felt he had lost the urge to empty his bowel, and that trips to the bathroom were now purely a matter of habit with little expectation of experiencing a satisfactory degree of rectal emptying. As it turned out, correcting his haemorrhoids depended totally on reversing his unfavourable toileting behaviour.

The main point of Brian's story is to emphasise the complex and initially subtle manner in which changes in our emotional and psychological circumstances can ultimately affect our bowel function. In turn, this can manifest as any number of different complaints – urgency and incontinence, constipation and bloating, straining and incomplete evacuation, haemorrhoids and pelvic floor pain.

I could cite literally hundreds of different cases from my practice of psychological and behavioural factors manifesting in hundreds of subtly different clinical presentations. What is probably more helpful, however, is to make the following general points, based on many years of clinical experience:

- In every case of altered bowel function, it is critical to first consider and, if appropriate, exclude the sorts of sinister diseases that we know can and occasionally do affect the bowel. These include colorectal cancer, ulcerative colitis, Crohn's disease, coeliac disease and other malabsorption syndromes. Basic blood tests and a colonoscopy are excellent first-line investigations where these serious conditions are being considered.

- Assuming that there is no longer any concern about the presence of a serious underlying bowel disorder, the role of psychological stress and/or behavioural factors in initiating or perpetuating the altered bowel function must be considered.

- Psychological and behavioural problems can also be caused by bowel dysfunction. Abnormal behaviour associated with the bowel symptoms might be the result of a bowel problem rather than the source of the problem. In some people, abnormal behaviour can be both cause and consequence of bowel dysfunction.

- All of this psychological and behavioural 'noise' can often create the impression that the problem is entirely psychological. As a result, it is all too easy to dismiss patients as being 'neurotic', and for this reason many patients don't get the most appropriate treatment either of their bowel symptoms or of their behavioural problems.

- Disciplined attention to the Three Golden Rules (see Chapters 3 and 4) and behavioural treatments such as The Three Ds (see Chapter 3) can be effectively introduced at the same time as more strictly medical treatments such as anti-diarrhoeal therapy, laxative treatment and even antidepressant or anti-anxiety medications. Non-medical behavioural therapies are critical elements of the effective management of many bowel disturbances, as well as of the problems they provoke.

9

Bowel problems in children

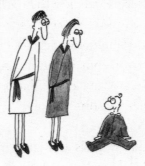

The vast majority of my patients are not children. I am not a paediatrician, so the views I express here about constipation in childhood – although strongly held – do not come with the same level of backing, drawn from extensive clinical experience, that my opinions about adults do. Nevertheless, I can make some general comments that might at least guide you in a helpful direction.

The transition from total social incontinence as an infant to independent continence as a toddler can be remarkably smooth or can turn into a battle of wits between child and parent that matches the Cold War.

Many factors play a part, and it is well beyond my area of expertise to outline them all here.

However, the inescapable conclusion for any child is that the emptying of their bowel seems to have a remarkably powerful impact on their parents – both on their parents' emotional state and, even more so, on the extent to which they become the focus of their parents' attention. In my opinion, this awareness – drawn from the child's experience during toilet training – rarely causes constipation, but it might serve to modify the child's responses to any constipation that might later develop for other reasons.

Just as for adults, girls are much more prone to constipation than are boys. But either sex can suffer during childhood from a painful anal fissure (a tear in the anal lining, resulting in intense pain and sometimes bright-red blood with the passage of a stool – see Chapter 2), and this is undoubtedly one of the most common, and most easily reversible, causes of childhood constipation.

A painful anus always needs proper medical assessment. Close inspection by an experienced doctor is usually all that is required (and appropriate) in the case of a child with an anal fissure. Treatment generally involves the use of non-habit-forming laxatives, which allow for softening of the stool, easing of the pain and, in many cases (unlike in adults), durable healing of the anal fissure. Lactulose syrup, macrogol powder (the tasteless version, which can be readily disguised in fruit juice) or liquid paraffin (especially the chocolate-flavoured version) may all be used in this situation.

Difficult problems with constipation generally only tend to begin when a child's bowel is unable to work for a more prolonged period, resulting in a degree of faecal impaction. Constipation might have started because of an inherent predisposition (such as in a girl) or as a result of a period of inadequate fluid or food intake, or a combination of both.

In this case, overstretching of the rectum and sigmoid colon can result, causing reduced ability of the bowel to sense the colorectal distension, and reduced force of propulsive colorectal muscular contractions. In short, a lower bowel that has become impacted with faeces can no longer sense when it is full, and has a markedly diminished ability to propel and expel its contents.

Furthermore, there is a tendency for softer faecal material to slip between the solid masses of constipated stool and to leak out of the anus, causing soiling and odour. This is referred to as 'overflow incontinence'. This incontinence is often passive and unconscious – the child literally has no feeling of the need to open their bowel and no capacity to control the leakage of soft faeces. Often, it is this incontinence that draws attention to the underlying impaction and constipation.

Initially, parents can be angry with their child, believing that they have suddenly become lazy in ignoring the urge to go to the bathroom to open their bowel and are simply doing it in their pants. Inevitably, parents also become frankly concerned. Apart from the offensive odour and the need for frequent clothing changes (not to mention quasi-industrial laundry services), they become anxious that their child will be ostracised by his or her peers, unable to participate in normal childhood activities and, not least, that there might be some serious and progressive underlying process that will require invasive correction.

Interestingly, some children in precisely this situation can be quite unmoved by their evidently unpleasant circumstances. There can be a form of secondary gain for the child as a result of attracting the undivided attention of their parents – especially given that the constipation itself is often not especially painful. I recall consultations with several children and their parents, the child sitting happily in my office and calmly watching the drama of his or her parents' distress play out.

So what can be done? Well, first and foremost it is important to ensure that the child (especially in the case of very little children) is having the right intake of food and fluid – constipation can be a reflection of inadequate food and/or fluid intake. Anal fissure and other painful perianal conditions also need to be considered and excluded.

In general, by the time I get to see (or hear about) these children, plenty of time has already passed, their diet has been considered and corrected, any anal fissure has been ruled out or treated and serious pathology is no longer a real consideration. At this stage, management of the chronically constipated child with faecal impaction – with or without overflow incontinence – is based on the following two simple principles:

1 *Get the bowel completely empty, and keep it empty.* Thorough, intermittent (weekly) bowel cleansing with a powerful osmotic laxative is exactly what these children require to completely empty their bowels, to eliminate the prospect of faecal soiling and to allow restoration of some spontaneous bowel activity. For children, I recommend an appropriate dose of a sweet osmotic sugar (lactulose, sorbitol) or the tasteless powder macrogol, dissolved in fruit juice or whichever liquid is easy to drink. As children become older and better able to cope with less palatable laxatives, all the usual osmotic agents (see Chapter 5) can be introduced.

2 *Reassure the parents that childhood constipation invariably improves as the child matures.* As children

enter their teens and early adolescence, they rapidly assume direct personal control for a problem that is, by now, a matter they no longer wish to share with their parents. The secondary gain that made them strangely indifferent to their own symptoms as young children inevitably disappears as they mature.

The overall approach, therefore, is to insist on a complete, once-weekly colonic emptying using a palatable (and safe) osmotic laxative, until either spontaneous colonic activity returns or the child (now entering their teens and adolescence) takes control of their own bowel affairs. Surgery should be regarded as the very last resort – in my experience, it is rarely appropriate for children.

10

Case studies

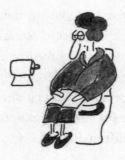

This chapter presents five real case studies from my practice (with names changed for privacy), to illustrate how some of the bowel problems discussed in earlier chapters can manifest and affect people's everyday lives – and how they can successfully be treated.

Case study 1:
Haemorrhoids and premature defecation

Mark was a 59-year-old retired policeman who had undergone numerous non–hospital-based treatments for his haemorrhoids at the hands of a number of different specialists for well over ten years. His haemorrhoids typically caused him to experience both bright-red rectal bleeding with almost every bowel action – on the toilet paper as well as dripping and spraying into the bowl on many occasions – as well as protrusion of his haemorrhoids with virtually every bowel action.

When I first saw him, Mark was opening his bowel up to five times every morning, accompanied by urgency and progressively more liquid stools as the morning went on. This was the typical pattern of what is often called 'irritable bowel syndrome'.

Because of the urgency associated with each bowel action, initiation of defecation was routinely prompt and effortless, occasionally even 'explosive'. However, because of the intense activity of his bowel and the liquid nature of his stools, he was rarely able to leave the bathroom quickly, sitting instead to wait for another contraction wave to bring down more stool, and wiping at length to clean up after what was an inevitably messy finish. With all the time he was spending in the bathroom – sitting and waiting and wiping and straining to finish that last little bit – Mark was a sitting duck for the development of haemorrhoids.

In the first instance, my objective was to reduce the amount of time and effort Mark was expending in the process of emptying his bowel. I prescribed a low dose of loperamide to be taken every morning and to be gradually increased every week or so until the desired stool frequency and consistency was achieved. Mark was thrilled that the solution to his haemorrhoids need not mean surgery or other potentially painful treatments, as had been his previous experience. He instituted the loperamide plan and returned to see me in three months.

On a dose of just 2mg of loperamide every morning, the frequency of Mark's bowel actions had decreased to just once or twice a day, and his stool consistency was significantly firmer; wiping up after a bowel action was now reliably quick and clean. More importantly, his bleeding had dramatically decreased ('by about 90 per cent') and all haemorrhoidal protrusion had been eliminated. Naturally, he was delighted with this improvement: he was more than happy to continue with this low dose of loperamide indefinitely. I reassured him about its absolute safety for long-term use at this dose, and discharged him from my care.

So far, Mark's story fitted nicely with my view that many haemorrhoids – especially those occurring in men (who are rarely constipated) – are caused by their over-active bowels and consequent need to spend lots of time in the bathroom. Likewise, his dramatic improvement with loperamide reinforced my strong belief in the importance of pursuing solid stool consistency to abbreviate the time spent in the bathroom.

But about three years later, Mark returned to see me complaining of passive soiling of soft stool occurring in the hour or so after his once-daily bowel action. His haemorrhoidal bleeding and protrusion had also begun to reappear, although nowhere near as prominently as previously. Mark was still using low-dose loperamide, but he had found that increasing the dose above 2mg daily in an attempt to further solidify his stool would result in his experiencing inordinate difficulty effecting rectal emptying. For this reason, he simply could not manage to achieve an appropriately solid stool consistency.

What was going wrong? Mark's reduced frequency to just one bowel action each morning was consistent with his regular use of the loperamide I had prescribed. But his recurrent haemorrhoidal symptoms suggested that he was once again spending more time and expending more effort in the bathroom. And his passive soiling of soft stool after defecation made it clear that not only was his stool consistency still too soft but he was continuing to experience incomplete rectal emptying. And why, when he increased his dose of loperamide – exactly as I had urged him to do – had he found that he struggled to open his bowel at all?

Further enquiry revealed the answer. I asked Mark precisely what prompted him to visit the bathroom each morning. After initially insisting that he did so because of a normal urge to go, he quickly conceded that he had always gone to the bathroom every morning, usually just after breakfast and with the newspaper in hand. However, since he had commenced taking loperamide years earlier, he now rarely initiated defecation promptly, and generally had to wait and even push a little to get things started. He then rarely felt completely empty, and often had to use a large amount of toilet paper to clean up what he described as soft and 'sticky' stool.

Mark was well aware that his stool consistency was still too soft. But when he increased his dose of loperamide, his regular morning bowel action would be even slower to get started and would regularly require him to strain; evacuation was even less complete (and even more frustrating) under these circumstances.

Even under the influence of a low dose of loperamide, Mark's bowel activity remained forceful and his stool consistency consequently soft. But his decision to visit the bathroom out of habit rather than in response to an appropriately forceful urge (a classic case of premature defecation) meant that he was not reaching the bathroom with a sufficiently strong urge to permit prompt and effortless initiation of defecation. In turn, he was also unable to achieve a satisfactory degree of rectal emptying, resulting in retention of stool after each bowel action with subsequent passive leakage of the retained stool (which was invariably still soft) after he left the bathroom.

In this situation, the solution for Mark rested not only with further firming of his stool consistency by a further increase in loperamide dosage, but with retraining him to only ever enter the bathroom with an appropriately strong urge. I outlined to him the importance of awaiting the arrival of an irresistible urge to go, and asked him to implement 'The Three Ds'. He was to delay visiting the bathroom until the urge was unequivocally strong; he was to leave the bathroom without straining if he found that he could not initiate defecation within 30 seconds; and he was to consciously distinguish between urges that resulted in prompt initiation of rectal emptying and those that simply left him sitting there wondering why he had decided to go in the first place.

I also implemented a blanket ban on all reading material being taken into the bathroom. If nothing happened quickly, he must not sit and read while awaiting the arrival of a contraction wave. There were to be no distractions from the job at hand – either he got the timing right and 'did his business' promptly, or he accepted that he had got it wrong and left the bathroom immediately.

When I next saw Mark two months later, he was taking 8mg of loperamide daily (two 2mg capsules, twice a day); this had eliminated leakage completely and had greatly reduced the amount of time he was spending in the bathroom. His haemorrhoidal symptoms had also disappeared. By delaying defecation until the urge to go was genuinely strong – by awaiting that irresistible urge – he had been able to achieve prompt and effortless initiation of defecation and brief and complete trips to the bathroom.

Interestingly, Mark had also found that he simply did not get the urge to go every single day: often it would be two days between bowel actions. He didn't mind this, as the extra time meant not only that he arrived with a reliably strong urge but that by then his stool consistency had become generally firmer and more solid. Mark claimed that the extra cost of loperamide was compensated for by using less toilet paper!

Mark's story, spread as it was over two separate periods of care, emphasises the following important points about both urge and stool consistency:

- Many people suffer from inherently overactive ('irritable') bowel function, and this can reliably be controlled with loperamide, often at low dosage.
- It is all too easy to get into the habit of making premature visits to the bathroom, without appreciating how this disconnects us from the all-important urge to go in the first place.

- Behavioural approaches to common conditions are often extremely effective, and can help us to avoid unnecessary or even futile surgery or other potentially unpleasant treatments.
- For many people, the ideal frequency is not once every day. Having a regular bowel action once a day is simply nowhere near as important as are the ease and the completeness of any individual bowel action.

Case study 2:
Slow colonic transit and speculative defecation

Brenda was a 54-year-old nurse who was first sent to see me because of troublesome perirectal pain (pain around the rectum). She had been seen by another surgeon, who had reassured her that no surgery was necessary. Instead she had been prescribed a local anaesthetic cream, with little benefit.

The pattern of Brenda's pain suggested an origin in the pelvic floor musculature. On more detailed enquiry, she described increasing difficulty with rectal emptying. As a general rule, she said, her bowel opened every day, and she described her stool consistency as 'normal'.

Nevertheless, Brenda had developed a progressively deteriorating pattern of straining at stool, with the ever-increasing awareness that she was unable to complete rectal evacuation. She found that she had to wait and 'relax' before her bowel would begin to work, and that she frequently needed to strain to keep things moving. Often, she experienced the sensation of a mechanical obstruction to the passage of stool, as if there was a narrowing or obstruction of the anal outlet.

Over time, Brenda had found that she would become uncomfortably aware of rectal fullness during the afternoon, and she had begun to visit the bathroom a second (and occasionally a third) time to try to empty her rectum and alleviate the discomfort. The discomfort of this rectal fullness and that of the perirectal aching became difficult to distinguish, but she rarely achieved a satisfactory degree of rectal emptying with these additional visits, which were almost invariably followed by genuinely distressing perirectal pain. There was mounting discomfort, confusion, frustration and upset.

On internal rectal examination, there was exquisite pelvic floor tenderness consistent with the impression of a muscular origin to her pain. But the cause of that muscular pain was the excessive straining in which she was engaging on a repeated basis. It was her pattern of rectal evacuation that was the root cause of her troubles.

I asked Brenda whether she ever experienced a strong urge to empty her bowel. In fact, she said, she hadn't experienced a genuine urge to do so for a number of years. But she also noted that, if she didn't go every day, she would rapidly become badly 'blocked up' and very uncomfortable indeed. On one occasion she had gone several days without opening her bowel; this had been frankly painful and had required laxatives by mouth and enemas to resolve. Following this unpleasant and undignified experience, Brenda had become fearful of ever repeating it in the future. Rather than risk such a repeat, she planned a visit to the bathroom every morning, after breakfast, to insist on a daily bowel action.

Brenda's difficulty with evacuation related to her decision to visit the bathroom before the arrival of an appropriately forceful urge. Her sensation of obstructed defecation was the result of paradoxical pelvic floor and external anal sphincter contraction (see Chapter 3), provoked by her intense voluntary straining. And her inability to effect complete rectal emptying was due to the combination of a genuinely inadequate propulsive urge and the angled, narrowed rectal outlet caused by her voluntary straining.

Brenda's trips to the bathroom every morning could be regarded as being 'pre-emptive', as she was obliging herself to empty her rectum, at least to some extent, even in the absence of any real urge to go. Her trips to the bathroom in the afternoon were better described as 'speculative', as she misinterpreted the discomfort associated with faecal residue in her rectum, combined with nagging pelvic floor soreness, as a genuine urge to go. Either way, Brenda was regularly and repeatedly reaching the bathroom and attempting to empty her rectum in the absence of any substantial urge.

But awaiting the irresistible urge was clearly not the answer in this case – Brenda had tried waiting for the arrival of a more forceful urge to evacuate but had found that this only seemed to compound her problems. Undoubtedly, she also suffered from a degree of slow colonic transit, whereby a forceful, spontaneous urge simply never appeared. In truth, Brenda no longer really knew when she should be going to the bathroom, and she had lost all confidence that there would be a worthwhile result when she did go.

The solution in Brenda's case required careful explanation of the various factors that were contributing to her problem – slow colonic transit, inadequate urge, and excessive voluntary straining. The first step in treatment was to reassure her that there was no fixed mechanical obstruction underlying her complaint, and therefore absolutely no need for surgical intervention. In short, the solution for Brenda rested with enhancing her colonic transit and modifying her toileting behaviour.

I recommended the introduction of a once-weekly laxative (I advised the use of magnesium sulfate in Brenda's case) taken at a sufficient dose to provoke a powerful urge and empty the bowel completely.

In turn, Brenda needed to consciously delay visiting the bathroom until the urge provoked by the large dose of magnesium sulfate was (almost) irresistible. This would enable her to initiate rectal emptying without the need for any straining and would ensure that, once the impact of the magnesium sulfate had subsided, she would be completely empty. In between weekly doses of magnesium sulfate, Brenda was not to use any other laxatives.

More importantly, I instructed Brenda in 'The Three Ds' (see Chapter 3) – she needed to:

- defer trips to the bathroom until the urge to go was compelling
- desist from sitting and straining in the bathroom if evacuation failed to commence within 30 seconds (or if it suddenly stopped midway), and
- distinguish between the sensations associated with prompt initiation of rectal evacuation (such as those provoked by a large dose of magnesium sulfate) and those that were nothing more than false alarms (such as those that had been prompting her regularly speculative visits to the bathroom in the afternoon).

Brenda's initial reaction was one of profound anxiety. She understood and accepted my explanation as to the cause of her symptoms and was, frankly, looking forward to the weekly clean-out. But the thought of waiting, possibly for six long days, until a strong urge arrived filled her with dread. All she could think about was that she would become incredibly blocked up if she was unable to get her bowel to work for that long.

I reassured Brenda that it would take her much longer than it had previously to become blocked up. Moreover, she would be able to resolve any degree of hold-up with her next weekly dose of magnesium sulfate. But I also appreciated that her anxiety was real and, rather than leave her to worry about it, I proposed a second dose of magnesium sulfate midweek in case she felt full and uncomfortable.

Brenda returned as planned two months later. She had managed to complete consecutive weekly clean-outs with magnesium sulfate, and had found that this definitely was associated with a strong urge and with complete emptying. However, she had found that she was still struggling to effect satisfactory rectal emptying during the week, and that she continued to sit and strain, convinced that she needed to empty her bowel but perplexed and discomfited by her inability to do so. Not surprisingly, she continued to be troubled by perirectal pain.

Despite experiencing a truly irresistible urge to evacuate (under the influence of a dose of magnesium sulfate), Brenda had been unable to override her longstanding habit of speculative trips to the bathroom. Even though the sensation that took her to the bathroom during the days between treatments with magnesium sulfate was unequivocally different from the powerful urge provoked by those treatments, the discomfort associated with the sensation of rectal fullness was proving too difficult for Brenda to ignore – she just had to see if she could gain relief by attempting to empty her bowel.

The good news, however, was that Brenda could now see much more clearly the folly of these speculative visits to the bathroom. On reflection, she appreciated how her faulty timing of trips to the bathroom was contributing to her need to strain, to her perirectal pain and to what was in fact an infuriating waste of her time. I pointed out to her that she had not become blocked up, despite her initial fears. I reiterated The Three Ds, and emphasised the importance of deferring any attempt at defecation until the sensation to evacuate was anything other than powerful. I urged her to test my treatment strategy by holding on throughout the week – unless, of course, a powerful need to evacuate spontaneously arose.

The next appointment was altogether briefer. Brenda had been able to apply The Three Ds between her weekly doses of magnesium sulfate, and had achieved the return of spontaneous and reasonably urgent bowel actions. These had been quite satisfactory, preceded by a good urge and associated with a comfortable degree of emptying. In the fortnight prior to this appointment, these spontaneous bowel actions had become a daily event, and Brenda had in fact begun to omit her strictly weekly doses of magnesium sulfate. Her pelvic floor pain was now almost inconsequential.

At the heart of all of Brenda's pre-emptive and speculative trips to the bathroom – the cause of her straining, her difficulty completing defecation and her pelvic floor pain – was her slow colonic transit and her own response to it. By restoring more normally brisk colonic transit, and by applying simple modifications to her toileting behaviour, she had been able to reverse the downward spiral of excessive straining and inefficient rectal evacuation. Her complaints, both physical and psychological, had in very large part been addressed.

Case study 3:
Soft stools, opportunistic defecation and faecal leakage

Joan was referred to see me because of her faecal incontinence. This was a deeply troubling problem for the 54-year-old divorcee, who had put her social life on hold because of her fear that episodes of incontinence would prove embarrassing and even 'fatal' to any new relationship. Having extricated herself from a long and unhappy marriage, and with her children now independent, she felt that she deserved the opportunity to explore some personal happiness.

The practical issue for Joan was that she experienced passive, unconscious leakage of faeces more or less throughout the day. This necessitated the wearing of a pad, and frequent pad changes due to soiling and staining. Leakage was likely to be most problematic when she went on her morning walk, regardless of how much time she had invested in emptying her bowel before heading off. She was anxious about the odour, and terrified at the prospect of leakage occurring during any intimacy with a new partner.

Joan also complained of difficulty with rectal emptying. She rarely experienced a strong urge to evacuate, and regularly left the bathroom feeling incompletely empty. Wiping up after a bowel action could be protracted, and often involved the use of excessive amounts of toilet paper. This was time-consuming and infuriating.

My first question for Joan was: How often did she open her bowel each day? Almost every time she sat down to empty her bladder. Did she go to the bathroom on those occasions with a strong urge to empty her bowel? Never. Were her bowel actions hard and difficult to expel? Quite the reverse – they were generally soft, unformed and paste-like in consistency.

When she was wiping up after a bowel action, the stool was soft and even sticky. What leaked out after a bowel action was equally moist and unformed. For Joan, the problem was one of passive leakage of stool that she simply could not expel during rectal evacuation.

As you will remember, the first and third Golden Rules for happy, healthy rectal evacuation emphasise the importance of reaching the bathroom with a strong urge to go and producing a solid, well-formed stool. The majority of Joan's attempts at evacuation were not associated with any preceding urge to do so but could better be described as 'opportunistic' – entirely secondary to her original intention, which was to empty her bladder. Similarly, Joan's stool consistency was invariably soft, rather than solid. Given the absence of any pressing urge to go, and given the unformed consistency of her stool, it was hardly surprising that she routinely failed to achieve complete rectal emptying.

The soft stool consistency and the evidently frequent filling of the rectum by faeces suggested that Joan's colonic transit was not unduly slow. So how could someone with apparently normal colonic transit be unable to achieve a strong urge to evacuate? And what could be done to correct these seemingly contradictory complaints?

Experience has taught me that attempting to firm the stool consistency in women can promptly create awkward constipation. Yet in women with urgency and even urge incontinence of soft stool, the use of loperamide can be every bit as important as it is in the treatment of these symptoms when they occur in men. However, the inherent female propensity to constipation is such that, in circumstances such as Joan's, all other aspects of toileting behaviour needed to be corrected before we could even consider implementing anti-diarrhoeal therapy.

In the first place, therefore, I recommended that Joan adhere to The Three Ds – this would be a process of behavioural retraining designed to allow her to rediscover the innate urge to defecate. The first step was to steadfastly desist from straining to empty her rectum whenever she sat down to pass urine and became aware of rectal filling. Likewise, she needed to ensure that she deferred, whenever possible, efforts to empty her bowel until the urge to do so was forceful – until there was 'clear and present danger' of having her bowel open. In desisting and deferring in this way, Joan would begin again to be able to distinguish between urges and sensations that would permit prompt and effortless initiation of rectal emptying and urges and sensations that would only result in the need to strain.

Joan was able to appreciate that her problem with completing rectal evacuation was central to her subsequent problems with faecal leakage. But she was sceptical that her problems with initiating rectal evacuation could be corrected by modifying her toileting behaviour. From her point of view, she was attempting to empty her bowel because she felt the need to do so and for no other reason. Moreover, she was anxious that consciously overriding the feeling of the need to empty her bowel would result in troublesome constipation – in becoming totally blocked and completely unable to empty anything at all. Simply put, Joan couldn't really see how she could 'desist' when that awkward feeling of rectal fullness was present.

To assist Joan in overcoming her fear of becoming bound up completely, I recommended the concurrent introduction of a daily soluble fibre supplement; in her case, psyllium husks. This would assist in rendering her stool consistency a little more formed and might even speed up colonic transit, thereby enhancing the arrival of a full-blooded urge. Meanwhile, I was able to reassure her that the additional fibre would not make her stool firmer – something that would only increase her fear of becoming constipated.

I asked Joan to return to see me in two months, by which time she had noticed some improvement.

Importantly, she had (mostly) been able to separate visits to the bathroom for bladder emptying from those for bowel emptying. This had resulted in much more satisfactory initiation of rectal evacuation on most occasions; she was still experiencing a sense of rectal fullness when she sat to pass urine, and occasionally she gave in to this sensation and strained to empty her bowel.

The introduction of psyllium husks had definitely helped to create more forceful urges to empty her bowel, but the consistency of her stools remained soft and leakage was still a significant problem. The time had come to more actively modify her stool consistency, and I recommended the gradual introduction of low-dose loperamide.

I prescribed loperamide at 0.33 mg per capsule (about one-sixth of the dose of a standard 'off the shelf' capsule), and asked Joan to take just one capsule every morning. Only after a whole week of daily loperamide, and only if her leakage remained problematic, was she to increase to two capsules daily. After another week she could increase the dose again if necessary, and continue to do so each week until she reached the desired impact on stool consistency and faecal soiling.

By the time Joan returned to see me after another two months, she had already contacted my office to request another prescription. She had settled on a daily dose of two capsules (a total of 0.66mg) and had found that this had eradicated her problem with soiling. She had stopped taking psyllium husks when her supply ran out but there had been no subsequent problems with either the initiation or the completion of defecation.

Joan was delighted. Her social confidence had been restored, and she was altogether more confident about initiating a new relationship. Her success had been the result of her application of those three Golden Rules for happy and healthy rectal evacuation – specifically, by adopting these important actions:

- resisting the feeling that she should be straining to evacuate her rectum when the urge to do so was evidently inadequate
- delaying trips to the bathroom for the purpose of emptying her bowel until the urge to do so was strong and true, and
- rendering her stool consistency solid by the judicious introduction of loperamide.

Case study 4: Urgency and incontinence

Bradley first came to see me with his mother. He was 22 years of age but was neither studying nor working. In fact, for more than seven years he had been living almost entirely at home, venturing out only rarely when it was absolutely essential. He had even had to complete his secondary school studies from home.

For as long as he could remember, Bradley had experienced a bowel habit characterised by frequent and urgent bowel actions. He could recall numerous episodes of urge incontinence occurring in public; these were distressing events during which he had minimal warning of the need to empty his bowel, accompanied by a frantic effort to locate and reach a public toilet. All too often, these episodes culminated in overwhelming urgency with frank incontinence of voluminous, liquid faeces; understandably, these were humiliating and deeply upsetting experiences.

On an average day at home, Bradley described three or four bowel actions, typically occurring in the morning after breakfast but also likely to occur after other meals. The first of each 'volley' of bowel actions tended to be the firmest and the easiest to control; the last was inevitably very loose, very urgent and generally the smallest in volume.

When he first came to see me, Bradley was taking no specific treatment, although he had been seen by a dietician on just one occasion. Unfortunately, the dietary advice he had been given had not had any immediate effect, and Bradley was simply too anxious about the possibility of being incontinent away from home to keep the follow-up appointment.

There was much more to Bradley's story than

simple urgency and incontinence. Appropriate investigations for the usual 'treatable' causes of diarrhoea – inflammation, infection, malabsorption and even thyroid disease – had long been completed without identifying a simple explanation. Undoubtedly, there were significant personality and behavioural problems that long predated his virtual confinement to home. In all likelihood, it was these behavioural problems and their management that had taken the medical focus away from his bowel and had resulted in what I regarded as an undeniably passive medical approach to the treatment of his bowel urgency.

Even Bradley's mother seemed to have come to accept the apparently untreatable nature of his bowel disorder, worn down (I imagined) by years of close involvement in all of his physical and mental health issues. It had been a relative of Bradley's, a retired medical practitioner, who had encouraged him to seek another opinion about the erratic workings of his bowel.

It had taken considerable courage on Bradley's part even to make it to the appointment to see me. His decision to venture beyond the safety of his home reflected his increasing sense of desperation about his bowel function and his life situation in general.

The pattern of Bradley's urgency – the volleys of ever-more-liquid and urgent stools, and its tendency to be at its worst away from home when his anxiety at the prospect of such urgency was likely to be at its greatest – strongly suggested a disorder of colonic motility, or so-called irritable bowel syndrome. Confident that there was no more serious underlying pathology, I recommended the introduction of regular oral loperamide.

Given the severity of his symptoms and the fact that he was male, I felt confident that he could commence at a daily dose of 2mg without risking constipation. I asked Bradley to take the same low dose every morning for one week before deciding whether it had been of any benefit. If it had, and if his urgency was under good control, he could continue at the same dose indefinitely.

But if that low dose was insufficient to eradicate urgency, he was to increase it to 4mg (two 2mg) every morning. Each week he was to decide whether the current dose was working to his satisfaction and, if not, to increase it further – to 6mg each morning, then to 4mg twice daily, then to 6mg twice daily and so on. The idea behind this gradual increase was simply to avoid suddenly provoking constipation, for fear that this would discourage Bradley from pursuing the strategy to its completion.

In Bradley's case, the impact of loperamide was prompt and dramatic. Within a few short weeks, he had figured out that he needed 6mg twice a day (a total of six 2mg capsules per day) to control his bowel habit, to eradicate urgency and to restore the simple confidence of being able to leave home at any time of the day free of the fear of being incontinent. Needless to say, both Bradley and his mother were delighted.

When I reviewed him after two months, I was able to reassure him about loperamide's absolute safety for long-term use at this modest dose – no systemic side effects, no interactions with his other medications and no tendency for the development of tolerance or addiction. In short, he could continue to use loperamide at the most effective dose indefinitely with total impunity. This he did, and on later follow-up for an unrelated surgical condition, I was able to confirm that he continued to take loperamide on a daily basis to almost complete effect.

One of the most striking and gratifying aspects of my practice over the past 25 years has been the manner in which people have had their lives transformed by the simple introduction of loperamide. Like putting a brake on a runaway cart, loperamide slows the speed of bowel function and restores control and social confidence for people suffering from colonic overactivity and all the miserable urgency and incontinence, anxiety and social isolation that it can cause.

Case study 5:
'Stool perception disorder' – a cautionary tale

Early on in my specialist practice, Anne was referred to me by her somewhat desperate family doctor because of progressively deteriorating constipation. At 46 years of age, this had been a problem for Anne for almost 20 years. She had demanded an appointment to see me despite her GP's reservations.

Certainly, Anne described great difficulty with her bowel. Without laxatives, she described complete inability to effect a bowel action. But even under the influence of laxatives, she found evacuation difficult to initiate and especially difficult to complete. It wasn't at all clear to me whether the principal problem was due to slow colonic transit or inefficient rectal emptying or a combination of the two. In the first instance, I recommended a trial of vigorous weekly bowel cleansing with magnesium sulfate.

On planned review two months later, Anne was clearly very distressed. She had found that the magnesium sulfate had provoked watery diarrhoea without delivering easier or more complete rectal emptying. From her perspective, she felt that she simply could not continue to cope with matters as they currently were. From my perspective, I felt uneasy about the degree of Anne's distress and her expectation that I should decide and act immediately.

I elected to arrange for her pattern of colorectal emptying to be assessed by the combination of a radioisotope colonic transit scan and a barium evacuation proctogram. The former revealed mildly delayed colonic transit, with hold-up principally in the descending colon. The latter revealed delayed initiation of rectal emptying but, ultimately, reasonably complete rectal emptying. The picture was that of mixed transit and evacuation disorders of generally mild severity only.

Just a matter of days prior to her next review appointment, Anne called me to say that she was in severe abdominal pain and that she hadn't had a bowel action for four days. I was confused and, frankly, a little frustrated at the disparity between Anne's symptoms and the lack of objective evidence of constipation. I directed her immediately to a nearby hospital emergency department for their independent assessment. A variety of tests was ordered there, the results of which proved normal.

Most importantly, an X-ray taken of Anne's abdomen was normal; there was no suggestion of intestinal obstruction and no evidence whatsoever of a build-up of faeces within her bowel. The X-rays looked, for all intents and purposes, like those of someone who had just enjoyed a perfectly satisfactory and complete bowel action.

When Anne came to see me for her planned appointment a few days later, her husband Don joined her for the first time. He was forceful, even angry, in his demand for a solution to his wife's deteriorating situation. Laxatives were clearly not the solution, according to Don. There had to be something else I could offer.

In retrospect, Don's insistence that I provide a solution to his wife's problem was more a reflection of his own frustration at Anne's despair and distress than a realistic expectation that I solve her problem. He just wanted her to be well and happy. In the face of their combined unhappiness, however, and reflecting my own inexperience at the time, I succumbed and offered Anne the prospect of extensive colonic resection in the hope of curing her constipation and alleviating her dismay. She gladly agreed, prepared to accept the very considerable risks of such surgery in search of a solution.

As it was, surgery proceeded smoothly. By the fifth post-operative day, Anne's bowel was working predictably frequently, with the nursing chart clearly recording the passage of loose stools virtually every two hours. I was relieved and pleased that there had been no serious technical complications, and asked Anne how it now felt to be having her bowel opened without the need to take any laxatives.

I have never forgotten Anne's response: 'Oh, I'm not having my bowels open – that's just water.'

That was the first time I appreciated how the stools that any individual produces can be sharply at odds with their own misguided expectations. In Anne's case, even well before her surgery, she failed to perceive the stools that she regularly passed as being suitable. Clearly, her expectation was that she should be producing stools of a quantity and a quality altogether different from what she was actually able to produce.

Anne interpreted the frequent and very loose stools that were the predictable and desirable result of her extensive bowel resection as being entirely unsatisfactory. In retrospect, the normal appearance of her abdominal X-ray despite her claim that she hadn't opened her bowel for four days could only be explained on the basis that she had simply failed to recognise the passage of stools during those four days for what it had been.

Anne's story left a strong impression on me. Her distress was real, but its cause arose primarily out of her disturbed perception of what her stools should look like. In reality, this was a psychological problem much more than one of altered intestinal physiology. The objective tests – the mild slow transit and slightly delayed rectal evacuation – were the reliable guides here. Surgery was technically successful, but failed to address the central problem in Anne's case.

Awareness of the profound interplay between psychological factors and bowel function extends to having an awareness of the manner in which an individual's psychological make-up can influence their perception and description of their bowel habits. For doctors caring for people with disturbed bowel function, the distress that their patients describe always needs to be measured against the objective abnormalities that can be reliably demonstrated on testing.

11

Frequently asked questions

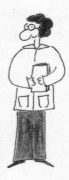

The following questions are some of those I have been asked frequently throughout my years of practice. I include them here as general guidance only. If you are unsure about any of the issues discussed here as they relate to your specific situation, please consult with your family doctor.

How do I know if I need to see my doctor?

If you are experiencing a problem with your bowel that is causing you discomfort, pain, inconvenience or worry, it is worth visiting your GP to see whether something can be done to alleviate this.

Almost the first thing any doctor will consider when a person presents with a bowel complaint is whether or not any serious bowel disease is likely to be present. The following symptoms and symptom patterns stand out as requiring more detailed investigation, to rule out pathologies such as cancer, polyps, infection and inflammation. If you have any of these, you should see your family doctor in order to rule out the possibility of serious bowel disease or, if disease is present, to have it treated promptly:

- *Bleeding from the bowel* Blood or blood-stained mucus, on the surface of or mixed in with stools, might suggest the presence of an underlying cancer, a large polyp or ulceration due to inflammation. Bleeding sufficient to cause iron deficiency or even anaemia (low haemoglobin level on blood testing) always requires more detailed investigation.
- *Change in your usual bowel habit* When a long-standing and predictable pattern of bowel function changes, concern is likely to be raised about the possibility of underlying bowel disease. This might be a change from regularity to unpredictability, or from a pattern of constipation to a pattern of loose stools (or the reverse). Recent onset of alternating constipation and diarrhoea may also suggest underlying bowel cancer.
- *Associated abdominal cramping* This might indicate a degree of bowel narrowing (possibly due to

bowel cancer) or the presence of either infection or inflammation.

- *Anal pain associated with bowel actions*   This is most often due to an anal fissure, but very occasionally might indicate a more serious condition such as an anal tumour or cancer.
- *Weight loss associated with bowel symptoms*   Recent and unplanned weight loss associated with bowel symptoms is always cause for concern.
- *Duration of symptoms*   Symptoms that have been present for less than six weeks might soon pass without event, while symptoms that have been present or intermittently present for 12 months or more tend to suggest a benign (non-serious) cause. However, symptoms that have been present for more than six weeks and have become progressively more insistent raise concerns about the presence of serious underlying pathology.
- *Symptoms occurring at night*   In the case of almost all benign bowel complaints, night-time and sleep are symptom-free times. Abdominal pain, diarrhoea and, especially, bloody diarrhoea occurring at night or waking you from sleep points to the presence of sustained and possibly serious underlying bowel disease.
- *Family history of serious bowel disease*   A family history of bowel cancer, ulcerative colitis or Crohn's disease raises additional concern where any of the symptoms listed above have developed.

In essence, if your symptoms include rectal bleeding and abdominal or anal pain, and if they have persisted and even progressed over six weeks or more, you must bring them to your doctor's attention. After a detailed assessment by your doctor, or where there is concern for any other reason, a colonoscopy (examination of the colon using a long, flexible telescope inserted through the anus) usually represents the most accurate means of detecting any serious bowel pathology. Your doctor will be well aware of the potential for serious pathology and will initiate appropriate investigation as required.

How do I know if I'm constipated?

Constipation means different things to different people. In an effort to provide some sort of standard definition, doctors often refer to the patient's stool frequency – how many bowel actions that individual has each day or each week – as the measure of normality. In general, a daily bowel action is regarded as normal, and having fewer than three bowels actions per week might be regarded as constipation.

However, recall the discussion in Chapter 1 about what constitutes 'normal'. It is true that people who are not constipated often open their bowels daily or even more frequently, while people who are unequivocally constipated often open their bowels less frequently than daily. But some people who open their bowels only once per week do so with ease and leave the bathroom feeling comfortably empty. Conversely, there are others who achieve only partial rectal emptying despite attempting to empty their bowels several times each day.

In reality, what makes someone constipated is not so much how often they open their bowel but how easily and completely they do so. Constipation is best regarded as being difficulty with either initiating or completing rectal evacuation. Common symptoms include weak and infrequent urges to go to the bathroom, straining to do so, requiring laxatives to achieve a bowel action, abdominal bloating and a sense of incomplete rectal emptying. If you are genuinely bothered by the difficulty you are experiencing in either starting or finishing a bowel action (or both), then I think that you can rightly describe yourself as constipated.

Shouldn't my bowel work naturally?

Yes, of course it should. Just like my cholesterol level should, naturally, be normal (rather than alarmingly high without medication). And just like somebody else's blood pressure should, naturally, not be raised to the point of needing medication.

The belief that our bowels should regulate themselves 'naturally' lies at the heart of the unfortunate and widespread reluctance to take the necessary medications that might speed up (or slow down) our malfunctioning intestines. Many people are completely convinced that the solution to their bowel problems must rest with diet and with diet alone (and, more often than not, with the ingestion of extra fibre).

This belief is misguided on three counts.

First, bowels malfunction just like any other part of the human body. They can be underactive or overactive or swing wildly between the two extremes. That they don't always work perfectly in every person on the planet seems to me entirely unremarkable. That they sometimes need medication for satisfactory management seems absolutely consistent with what we all know about the human body and its all-too-frequent failings.

Second, diet alone cannot resolve the full range of our potential bowel problems any more than it can resolve the full range of our other health problems, such as high cholesterol, high blood pressure, diabetes and so on. Dietary manipulation forms an important element of the treatment of all sorts of health problems, including problems with bowel function, but it is rarely the whole answer. And in many cases increasing dietary fibre intake can aggravate rather than improve your bowel symptoms.

Third, the medications that so many of us do need to take to maintain comfortable control over our bowels are mostly extremely safe and entirely suitable for long-term use. Loperamide for those with loose stools and osmotic laxatives for those with constipation have minimal absorption into our bloodstream, meaning that they have very few side effects outside the intestines themselves. And they are not habit-forming, meaning that you can continue to take them for as long as they are working, confident that the current dose is likely to continue working without ill effect.

My husband tells me I need to eat more fruit, but eating more fruit doesn't work for me. Why not?

As a general rule, men have faster colonic transit than women, along with reliably frequent bowel actions accompanied by reliably strong urges to evacuate their bowels. (Recall from Chapter 2 that boys and men are generally 'good bowel athletes'.) Men also tend to respond briskly to any food or medication that speeds up colonic transit. Conversely, women are prone to having slow and sluggish bowels, and to being especially sensitive to any medications that slow bowels down (see Chapter 4).

Many men have an annoying tendency to parade their bowel athleticism in front of their inherently less (bowel-)athletic female partners. Simplistically, he concludes that if eating extra fruit and vegetables makes *him* go more often and more easily, then surely eating extra fruit and vegetables will do the same for *her*. But it's just not that simple.

For women with slow colonic transit, the laxative action of fruits, vegetables and fibre more generally is particularly weak. Even a massive increase in dietary fibre intake often fails to move a determinedly sluggish colon. Yet, even in this sluggish colon, bacteria reside appropriately in their billions and act on all this undigested dietary fibre to form unwanted excess gas (flatus).

Abdominal bloating, not infrequently painful, is thus a characteristic complaint among patients with slow transit constipation. And this bloating is largely due to the distension of their colon by flatus, which their sluggish colon produces quite normally but cannot adequately propel and expel. By increasing their dietary fibre intake, women with slow colonic transit routinely experience an undesirable increase in bloating far in excess of any desirable speeding up of colonic transit.

So you can tell your husband that he is welcome to increase his fruit intake whenever he feels the need. You can also tell him that what works for him may not, alas, work for you. The fact that you don't find eating more fruit helpful to your constipation – or that it actually makes your tendency to abdominal bloating worse – is quite consistent with your being a woman.

Shouldn't I be taking laxatives every day? I'm frightened I'll become too constipated if I don't open my bowel at least once a day.

The belief that our bowels should work every day is deeply embedded in our society. But, as discussed in Chapter 1, what matters much more than having a bowel action every day is that our bowel actions are, as much as possible, prompt and effortless, brief and complete. How often we open our bowels is simply nowhere nearly as important as how easily and completely we do so. To this end, the weekly (not daily – see Chapter 5) use of an effective dose of laxatives can assist.

Many people – mostly women (see Chapter 2) – do not need to open their bowels every day. They can safely and very comfortably wait until they experience a spontaneous – and appropriately forceful (see Chapter 3) – urge to open their bowels before doing so. If such an urge takes several days to develop, that is absolutely fine. If no such urge arrives after a whole week, it is totally safe and appropriate to clean out thoroughly by taking another decisive dose of laxatives.

While a bowel habit characterised by laxative-induced cleansing once a week (with few or even no spontaneous bowel actions in between) is an undeniably foreign concept, it is nevertheless absolutely safe and sustainable. In fact, it is far better to clean out thoroughly just once per week with a substantial dose of laxatives than it is to effect incomplete evacuation day after day as a result of the daily use of smaller doses.

How can I hold on until the urge to go is 'irresistible'? Whenever I delay going when I think I need to, I end up not being able to go at all.

In a perfect world, every one of us would be able to regularly and reliably generate an 'irresistible' urge – provided we have waited long enough for that urge to arrive – that would predictably and satisfactorily empty our bowels. The truth, however, is that many people (mostly women) have inherently sluggish colonic transit and only rarely, if ever, experience a forceful urge to empty their bowels.

Many of these people have, therefore, learnt to recognise what represents the 'best' urge they are likely to experience, and respond to that sensation by heading to the bathroom. They have also learnt that they are likely to have to strain to initiate evacuation, and that they might not feel completely empty when they leave the bathroom. They know from experience that it is far better to respond to the 'best' urge than it is to wait in hope for something stronger – which, deep down, they know is never going to arrive. If they miss this opportunity, they have come to know, they are likely to become genuinely impacted and uncomfortable, and will likely need to take laxatives to correct the situation.

This need to respond to a modest urge – precisely because an irresistible urge is unlikely ever to appear – is the characteristic pattern of slow colonic transit. It represents a clear signal that steps should be taken to speed up (and, hopefully, restore speedier, spontaneous) colonic transit. In this circumstance, the regular or intermittent use of an osmotic laxative (see Chapter 5) is definitely the way to go.

How can I tell whether the urge to go is real or just a 'false alarm'?

One of the most difficult challenges I face in looking after people with evacuation disorders is trying to explain the notion of a false or misleading urge to empty their bowels. People in this situation find it genuinely confusing when I ask them to explain what it is that makes them choose to attempt to evacuate their bowels at any given point in time. Why else would anyone try to empty their bowel if not in the belief that they needed to do so then and there?

But very many people do enter the bathroom with an inadequate urge to empty their bowels, notwithstanding their strong conviction (and ardent hope) that that is what they need to do. In truth, for many people, the feeling of needing to evacuate their bowels is not accompanied by any confidence that successful evacuation will ensue. Rather, despite the compelling sense of needing to go, they more often than not arrive in the bathroom correctly anticipating difficulty, discomfort and frustration.

When I am talking with such a patient, I ask whether they have ever either experienced some form of gastroenteritis or undergone a colonoscopy (each of which brings on overwhelming diarrhoea with urgent and watery stools). Nearly every patient I see has experienced one or the other of these at some point in their life. When I ask them to recall that urgent call to evacuate their bowel and to compare it to the feeling that more usually prompts them to attempt evacuation, the distinction is readily apparent.

An absolutely routine question to my patients is: 'When you go to the bathroom to open your bowel, is it in response to an irresistible urge to go at that instant?' Under this sort of direct enquiry, most people concede that they are able to tell the difference between the real thing and a false alarm.

A related question, also totally routine in my practice, is 'When you sit on the toilet, does your bowel action commence immediately, or do you have to wait or strain to get things started?' Failure to promptly and spontaneously initiate a bowel action is cogent evidence that your decision to sit on the toilet at that moment was flawed, that the urge to empty your bowel was inadequate or misleading. If you regularly fail to commence rectal evacuation within just 30 seconds of sitting on the toilet, you are almost certainly choosing to attempt evacuation in the absence of a sufficiently strong urge to go.

Isn't it better for stools to be soft?

In general, the quicker the colonic transit, the softer the stool is likely to be, and the more urgent will be the need to empty your bowel. Consequently, initiation of rectal evacuation in this situation is likely to be easy.

However, if colonic transit is too quick, stools can become excessively liquid and pressingly urgent to pass, even to the point of provoking urge incontinence of faeces. Moreover, although soft and fast-moving stools do make the initiation of defecation easy, they can also make it extremely difficult to achieve complete rectal evacuation, since even unusually powerful intestinal contraction waves tend to fade and disappear before the stool has been completely passed. So, despite being associated with a promisingly strong urge to go to the bathroom, soft faeces can all too easily be left behind after defecation, leaving with it an acute and uncomfortable awareness that the rectum has not been emptied.

The truth is that the ideal stool consistency for satisfactory and complete rectal evacuation is firm and well formed (see Chapter 4). Provided that it is accompanied by a strong and true urge to initiate rectal evacuation, a firm and well-formed stool is unequivocally optimal for the completion of rectal evacuation.

Speedy colonic transit undoubtedly favours easy initiation of defecation, while firm and well-formed stool consistency undoubtedly enables complete rectal emptying. The trick is to balance the pursuit of the ideal stool consistency with consciously deferring rectal evacuation until the urge to do so is strong.

Is it better to use moist wipes or plain toilet paper?

This is a real 'First World' conundrum! Nevertheless, it is a genuine one, since many people do use moist wipes rather than toilet paper, and many of those who do genuinely believe that it is the healthier alternative.

Before answering this question, it is worth noting that the perianal skin (the skin around the anus) in human beings likes to be clean and dry. You might well ask yourself, if human perianal skin is so concerned about being clean and dry, why did it position itself in an area so prone to moisture and soiling? This human design enigma notwithstanding, the undeniable truth is that perianal skin that is moist and/or soiled is prone to become broken, chafed or overtly macerated, which can result in stinging, itching, burning pain and even bleeding.

So leaving the bathroom after a bowel action with our perianal skin clean and dry is absolutely what we want. But when our stools are soft and sticky, we often find it difficult to wipe up completely. Repeated wiping is time-consuming, frustrating and, not infrequently, a little painful. In these situations, a moist wipe makes the process of cleaning up quicker and more comfortable.

But moist wipes are, well, moist! By their very definition they generally do not leave the skin dry. (Their use should therefore really be followed by gentle drying with soft toilet paper.) Further, many moist wipes also contain soaps and scents that might irritate the skin of sensitive individuals. For these reasons – residual moisture and chemical sensitivity – moist wipes are not always as suitable and straightforward a solution as they might first seem.

The real 'trick' to getting the perianal skin clean and dry has nothing to do with the material with which we choose to wipe the area. A firm and well-formed stool that is accompanied by a genuinely strong urge to evacuate will almost always pass completely, leaving nothing behind within the rectum and no residue on the skin. Almost every person I have ever spoken to about the workings of their bowels can recall the passage of precisely such a well-formed, solid stool (even if it was a long time ago), and can remember fondly the accompanying sense of complete rectal emptying, snug anal closure and perianal cleanliness.

So the best way to keep your perianal skin clean and dry is to keep your stool consistency firm and well-formed. Moist wipes are almost always only necessary where stool consistency is too soft.

Why do I find it so difficult to go to a public toilet to open my bowel?

This is a common grievance. Very few people are completely at ease sharing the workings of their bowels with anyone at all – even close family, let alone total strangers. The sounds and smells, especially, of our bowels at work are matters of utmost privacy to all but a tiny percentage of the human population. And public toilets – a little like the public ablution blocks of Ancient Rome – are remarkably public places. It is not at all surprising, then, that many people find it awkward and embarrassing to open their bowels in this environment, and that they will therefore avoid this situation as much as they possibly can.

Given this deep and widespread reluctance to embark upon a bowel action in a public toilet, the likelihood is high that you will only go in public when the urge is truly irresistible. In other words, having done your level best to defer defecation until you get to a private facility (preferably in your own home), it is generally only when you have little choice that you will go in public. At least then you can be assured that the strength of the urge is likely to provide excellent impetus to favour prompt and effortless initiation and complete evacuation.

Deferring defecation until you can be at ease and free of embarrassment is completely acceptable. We have anal sphincters to close off the anus, and our rectum has the physiological capacity for 'receptive relaxation' (see Chapter 2) precisely for the purpose of 'holding on' when it is inconvenient or even dangerous to stop and open our bowels.

As long as, having delayed that trip to the bathroom until a more private opportunity presents itself, you await the arrival of another forceful urge to empty your bowel, you should be fine. As discussed in Chapter 3, sitting on the toilet waiting for a bowel action to start just because you had the urge a few hours earlier is a form of speculative defecation, and is a recipe for straining and frustration. If you do choose to hold on and not go when the urge is strong, just make sure you await the arrival of the next strong urge before attempting to open your bowel.

I've been told I have lactose intolerance. Should I see a dietician?

The short answer is: why not? An appropriately experienced dietician will review your current diet and adjust it according to your specific requirements.

There is much public awareness nowadays about dietary sensitivity to things such as gluten (a protein found in wheat, barley, rye, oats, spelt and other grains), lactose (found primarily in dairy products) and FODMAPs (sugars contained in a vast range of fruits, vegetables and grains). Accordingly, there are any number of 'exclusion diets' that can be applied in an effort to control troublesome gastrointestinal symptoms.

A comprehensive discussion of these dietary sensitivities is beyond the scope of this book. Certainly, in my opinion, these diets should only be conducted under the supervision of a qualified dietician. I will also make these two brief points:

• Dietary sensitivities are frequently postulated – by friends, relatives, even pharmacists, dieticians and doctors – but rarely confirmed or proven. Many, many more people embark on exclusion diets than are ever actually helped by them.

• The deep reluctance among the general population to resolve gastrointestinal symptoms by using medications – even simple, essentially innocuous ones like loperamide or osmotic laxatives – drives people to attempt dietary manipulation that can be unhealthy, profoundly unpalatable and often utterly useless. Symptom relief is often achieved more quickly, with less self-deprivation and misery, and in a manner that permits the maintenance of a genuinely healthy and balanced diet by the use of medications.

I've been advised to rest my feet on a low stool when I'm opening my bowel. Will this help?

Having our hips flexed – sitting on the toilet with our knees slightly higher than our hips – serves to relax the pelvic floor muscles and help open the anorectal outlet (see Chapter 3, and especially Figure 3). This is why the vast majority of toilets are lower than the standard sitting chair. For people who find that they need to strain to initiate or complete rectal evacuation, additionally flexing their hips assists this process further.

But the essential problem is rarely, if ever, the posture. Rather, it is the absence of a sufficiently strong urge. I have looked after scores of people who experience overwhelming urgency and outright urge incontinence of faeces while, bolt upright, they are running to find a bathroom. They certainly didn't need to have their hips flexed to get their bowels working. Conversely, I have treated scores more patients who have been bedevilled by a sense of obstructed defecation regardless of the posture they adopt, because they have attempted defecation in the absence of an appropriate urge. No degree of squatting ever helped them.

I have nothing against the little stools and footrests that people do use, and I appreciate that they make a big difference for some people. But the urge to go – or the lack thereof – is nearly always the critical issue, and not the posture adopted on the toilet. If you are able to get to the bathroom with an urge that is strong and true, you will be able to initiate defecation promptly and effortlessly without the need for any kind of furniture to modify your posture.

Epilogue

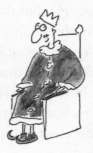

As easy as it is to dismiss or even laugh at the problems people experience with their bowels, what is absolutely undeniable is that, at every minute of every day in every corner of the planet, many people's bowels are causing them considerable concern and distress. Although disturbances of bowel function are often the result of genuine and sometimes serious pathology, an awful lot of the bowel-related trouble we human beings experience is the result of factors that can be modified and corrected very simply.

I have found over my years of clinical practice that the best way to understand and treat the malfunctioning bowel is to closely observe the well-functioning bowel and to identify what it is that accounts for such good and satisfactory function. As I have stressed throughout this book, every satisfactory bowel action is unambiguously prompt and effortless, brief and complete. And as I have also stressed, such satisfaction may be achieved by observing the three Golden Rules: consciously delaying trips to the bathroom until the urge to do so is pressing; diligently banishing reading material, electronic devices and any other distracting influences from the bathroom; and maintaining a firm and well-formed stool consistency.

For people prone to somewhat overactive bowels and consequently soft stool consistency, I frequently recommend the introduction of the anti-diarrhoeal medication loperamide. Even at low doses, this agent can have a life-changing effect on people suffering the consequences of loose stool with incomplete emptying and subsequent soiling.

Conversely, for those with inherently sluggish bowels – most often women – speeding things up is an almost certain prerequisite for achieving more satisfactory evacuation. I strongly favour osmotic laxatives of the 'salt' variety, taken infrequently but at effectively cleansing doses.

For many people experiencing an unsatisfactory bowel habit, the usual connection between the sensation of the need to go and the timing of our trips to the bathroom has become entirely severed. Trips to the bathroom for these individuals can be somewhat premature, overtly pre-emptive or anxiously speculative. In each case, these people reach the bathroom with an urge that is weak, absent or frankly misinterpreted.

As a result, in attending to almost every individual with disordered rectal evacuation, some focus needs to be applied to correcting the behavioural elements that form part – sometimes a very large part – of the problem. Delaying visits to the bathroom until the urge is strong and true, leaving the bathroom if evacuation has not started promptly (rather than hanging around and struggling) and relearning to distinguish between genuine urges and false alarms comprise a simple but effective set of behavioural strategies in cases of faulty rectal evacuation.

Only when the bowel is empty do we feel truly comfortable. The unequivocal objective of every single bowel action is to achieve complete emptying of the lower bowel. An empty bowel is a happy bowel, and this is optimally achieved by combining a powerful urge to empty the bowel with a solid and well-formed stool.

When all is said and done, however, it is our ability to reach the bathroom with an unequivocally powerful urge to empty our bowel that is the single most important element of a truly satisfactory bowel habit.

And it is the failure to either generate or await the arrival of such an urge that is most likely to result in a problematic and deeply disheartening bowel habit. Urge really is king.

Appendix

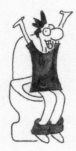

The four key characteristics of a satisfactory bowel action

Every truly satisfactory bowel action has four things in common – it is:

- prompt
- effortless
- brief, and
- complete.

The three Golden Rules of happy, healthy rectal evacuation

To achieve a bowel action that is prompt and effortless, brief and complete, we must observe the following three critical Golden Rules:

- **Golden Rule Number One:** Never attempt to empty your bowel until the urge to do so is strong and true.
- **Golden Rule Number Two:** Never, ever, take any distracting influences – newspapers, books, magazines, mobile devices – with you to the bathroom.
- **Golden Rule Number Three:** The ideal consistency for a human stool is solid.

The Three Ds

The Three Ds refers to the following simple behavioural approach to correct the faulty toileting behaviour associated with 'speculative defecation:

- **Defer** Speculative defecators must make a conscious decision to *defer* visiting the bathroom until the urge to go is strong and true.
- **Desist** When rectal evacuation does not commence both promptly and effortlessly, rather than sit and strain, the speculative defecator must *desist* – they need to get up and leave the bathroom immediately.
- **Distinguish** Developing the ability to *distinguish* between real urges and false alarms is the essence of correcting speculative defecation and its associated problems of straining, haemorrhoids and pelvic floor pain.

Glossary

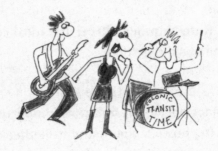

anal fissure a split or tear in the lining of the anus, at the junction between inside and outside

anorectal outlet the rectum and anal canal, through which faeces is expelled

anus (*also* **anal canal**) the short, final component of the large intestine

ascending colon the right side of the colon, immediately beyond the caecum

bowel in medical terminology, synonymous with intestine; in everyday language, refers to the large intestine

caecum the first part of the large intestine

colon the first and longest part of the large intestine; comprises the caecum, the ascending colon, the transverse colon, the descending colon and the sigmoid colon

colonic lavage a commercially available rectal irrigation technique administered by registered nurses

colonic transit time the time it takes faeces to move through the large intestine, from entering the caecum to being expelled through the anus

colonoscopy examination of the colon using a long, flexible telescope inserted through the anus

defecation the act of emptying the bowel

descending colon the left side of the colon joining transverse and sigmoid colon

faecal impaction when a hard mass of stool becomes stuck in the bowel due to chronic constipation

faeces the contents of the large intestine

flatus the gas passed out of the large intestine

insoluble fibre fibre found in foods that remain crunchy even when placed in liquid (nuts, fruit peel and pulp, many vegetables); this type of fibre tends to be more stimulating to our bowels than soluble fibre, and encourages softer stools

large intestine (*also* **large bowel**) starts where the small intestine ends; comprises the colon, the rectum and the anus

lavage *see* colonic lavage

mass movements muscle-contraction waves that propel faeces through the colon

overflow incontinence of faeces in cases of severe constipation, a tendency for softer faecal material to slip between or around the solid masses of constipated stool and leak out of the anus

perianal skin the skin around the anus

peristaltic (of muscle contractions) wave-like

pre-emptive defecation obliging one's bowel to work when there is no natural urge to do so

premature defecation anticipating the working of one's bowel when the urge is still some way off

rectal irrigation the instillation of warm tap water into the rectum to effect rectal emptying

recto-anal inhibitory reflex a reflex that relaxes the internal anal sphincter muscle when faeces descends into the lower rectum in anticipation of imminent evacuation

rectum part of the large intestine, approximately 12 cm in length, joining the colon to the anus

sigmoid colon the last component of the colon, usually a tortuous segment joining the descending colon to the rectum

small intestine (*also* **small bowel**) starts where the stomach ends and continues until the large intestine begins

soluble fibre fibre found in foods that are soft and that soften further when soaked in liquid (bran, porridge, psyllium husks); this type of fibre tends to encourage bulky and well-formed stools

speculative defecation attempting to defecate in response to a sensation that is not a true and pressing urge

stool the faeces passed out during a bowel action

stool frequency the number of bowel actions an individual has in a given period of time – per day or per week

transverse colon the central component of the colon joining the ascending and descending colon

urge incontinence of faeces inability to control the sudden urge to evacuate stools that have become excessively liquid and pressingly urgent to pass

Index

Acknowledgements

I am indebted to the staff of Fremantle Press who have brought this book to publication. My particular thanks go to Georgia Richter whose appreciation of its intention and whose positivity breathed life into the project; and to Leila Jabbour who, in greatly enhancing the initial manuscript, displayed an appreciation of the subject matter far beyond reasonable expectation.